VIOLENCE IN AMERICA

VIOLENCE IN AMERICA

A Public Health Approach

EDITED BY

MARK L. ROSENBERG
MARY ANN FENLEY

New York   Oxford
OXFORD UNIVERSITY PRESS
1991

Oxford University Press

Oxford   New York   Toronto
Delhi   Bombay   Calcutta   Madras   Karachi
Petaling Jaya   Singapore   Hong Kong   Tokyo
Nairobi   Dar es Salaam   Cape Town
Melbourne   Auckland

and associated companies in
Berlin   Ibadan

Published by Oxford University Press, Inc.,
200 Madison Avenue, New York, New York 10016

Oxford is a registered trademark of Oxford University Press

Library of Congress Cataloging-in-Publication Data
Violence in America : a public health approach /
edited by Mark L. Rosenberg and Mary Ann Fenley.
p. cm.
Consists of the revised papers from
the Surgeon General's Workshop on
Violence and Public Health,
held Oct. 27-29, 1985 Leesburg, Va.
Includes bibliographical references and index.
ISBN 0-19-506437-2
1. Violence—United States—Congresses.
2. Family violence—United States—Congresses.
3. Crime prevention—United States—Congresses.
4. Public health—United States—Congresses.
5. Victims of crimes—Medical care—United States—Congresses.
I. Rosenberg, Mark L., 1950- .
II. Fenley, Mary Ann.
III. Surgeon General's Workshop on Violence and Public Health
(1985 : Leesburg, Va.)
[DNLM: 1. Public Health—congresses. 2. Violence—congresses.
BF 575.A3 / V7945 1985] HN90.V5V5325 1991
303.6′0973—dc20 DNLM/DLC for Library of Congress
90-14341

1 2 3 4 5 6 7 8 9

Printed in the United States of America
on acid-free paper

Foreword

Throughout our history, Americans have remained committed to a social contract that respects the rule of law, that promotes peaceful intercourse among citizens, and that has as its highest value the protection of human life. We are often characterized as being a "violent nation" and clearly we have had some unpleasant chapters in our long history of nation building. Yet the values passed down to us through the years have consistently been the values of a people devoted to peace and the veneration of life.

Our citizens want to live in peace, but each year many thousands of them become the victims of violence. Some are infants, others are elderly and frail. They are abused, beaten, raped, assaulted, and killed. Society has somehow failed them. But such an admission must not be the end of the matter; for those of us in the health professions, that failure signaled the need for a new beginning. The Surgeon General's Workshop on Violence and Public Health, conducted in October 1985, represented that new beginning and encouraged all health professionals to respond constructively to the ugly facts of interpersonal violence.

Identifying violence as a public health issue is a relatively new idea. Traditionally, when confronted by the circumstances of violence, the health professions have deferred to the criminal justice system. Over the years we have tacitly and, I believe, mistakenly agreed that violence was the exclusive province of the police, the courts, and the penal system. To be sure, those agents of public safety and justice have served us well. But when we ask them to concentrate more on the prevention of violence and to provide additional services for victims, we may begin to burden the criminal justice system beyond reason. At that point, the professions of medicine, nursing, and the health-related social services must come forward and recognize violence as their issue and one that profoundly affects the public health.

As the chapters in this volume amply demonstrate, this is an awesome challenge to the health profession, but it is not totally uncharted. For some time, a number of people around the country have been doing the research and conducting pilot demonstrations to further engage the health professions in this issue of interpersonal violence. From the time of the workshop in 1985 to now, the exploration of effective means of public health intervention into elder abuse and child abuse, rape and sexual assault, spouse abuse, child sexual abuse, and assault and homicide has continued to grow. I look forward to continued progress in this area that is of such great significance for the health and well-being of all Americans and of our society as a whole. It will be a major contribution toward the strengthening of our nation's social contract.

C. Everett Koop, M.D., Sc.D.
Former Surgeon General
Public Health Service

Preface

The authors of the chapters in this book have much to tell you about the problem of violence, its importance, and impact. I will instead make a few observations about how violence compares with other public health problems and what we can learn from our public health experience regarding how to pursue the problem of violence.

AN HISTORICAL PERSPECTIVE

Throughout history, the two leading causes of early or premature death have been infectious diseases and violence. Infectious disease control started in 1796 with the work of Edward Jenner when he developed the first vaccine—for smallpox. Infectious disease control continued along with many nonspecific social changes, such as better nutrition, better housing, and education. In the past fifty years, we have returned to some specific tools, including vaccines, antibiotics, and pesticides.

In contrast, violence has defied the best minds in health, politics, religion, and law enforcement, and therefore has often appeared to be inevitable. This and other forms of fatalism must be actively opposed. That we live in a cause-and-effect world is as true with violence as with infectious diseases, an important observation for both public health people and educators.

Another important observation is that public health is in the business of continually redefining the unacceptable. This changes the social norm, which in turn changes the problem. For example, some forty years ago, polio was the inevitable price of summer in the United States. With the widespread use of polio vaccine in the 1960s, the social norm in this country quickly changed. However, for the hemisphere as a whole, the social norm has been polio control or relatively low levels of polio disease. When the regional director of the Pan American Health Organization announced that polio would be eliminated from this hemisphere by 1990, that one announcement changed the social norm, and it instantly became unacceptable to have any cases of polio in the Western Hemisphere.

From such experiences we can see how important it is to redefine the unacceptable in interpersonal violence. It becomes a major step in enlisting the public health structure of this country in changing the social norm. It should be understood that many have seen violence as being unacceptable just as many saw polio as being unacceptable. But until recently, violence has not been regarded as a public health problem. Rather, it has been viewed as a law enforcement problem, or as a transportation problem, or as a welfare problem. Dr. Koop is largely responsible for putting this on the public health agenda.

RECENT DEVELOPMENTS

In 1977 a group began looking at morbidity and mortality in the United States to advise on the twelve most important things that could be done in prevention. They made popular the notion of not only looking at the leading causes of death but also looking at the leading causes of years lost before age sixty-five. Heart disease, cancer, and stroke lead the list of causes of death, but the leading causes of years lost prematurely are injuries, cancer, heart disease, homicide, and suicide. They showed that three of the five leading causes of premature death—injuries, homicide, and suicide—are related to violence. It was because of this finding that the Centers for Disease Control started a program of violence epidemiology and hired Dr. Mark Rosenberg, who had training in both psychiatry and epidemiology, to head that program.

In 1979 the surgeon general published his book, *Healthy People*, outlining the fifteen priority areas requiring national attention in prevention. In 1978 the first meetings of health people from around the country were held to develop the 1990 objectives, a set of over 220 specific objectives pointing to where the United States should be in health by 1990. These include specific objectives on homicide rates, child abuse rates, and suicide, as well as on specific risk factors. This national prevention strategy is a landmark in public health, and it is important that violence is a part of the strategy.

In 1985 the National Academy of Sciences and the Institute of Medicine published *Injury in America—A Continuing Public Health Problem*. It pointed out that injury, both intentional and unintentional, remains the major unaddressed public health problem of our day. Whereas injury accounts for 4.1 million years of life lost before age sixty-five each year, heart disease and cancer combined account for only 3.8 million years lost before age sixty-five. Yet we spend $1.622 billion per year on research for the latter and only seven percent of that amount on injury research.

Basic to every successful public health effort has been the development of an appropriate surveillance system. This was true of the public health pioneers, such as Jenner, Snow, and Semmelweiss, who did limited but rigorous surveillance of a microcosm; but it is also true of the institutional pioneers who have developed surveillance of cities, provinces, and then entire countries.

The first nationwide surveillance system for any disease in this country was instituted only in 1950. That system was developed for malaria and made the startling discovery that indigenous malaria had quietly disappeared from this country some time in the 1940s without being noticed. We did not organize another nationwide surveillance program for five more years. In 1955 because of a problem with polio vaccine that still contained virulent virus, a nationwide poliomyelitis surveillance program was launched, literally overnight.

Global surveillance for a disease was not developed until the late 1960s as part of the smallpox eradication program. Although it may appear late to develop violence surveillance programs, in fact, surveillance in general is in its infancy.

Surveillance is essential if there is to be a concerted effort in violence control. We must define all aspects of the problem, collect relevant and correct data, analyze that data in order to define interventions, and measure the impact of those interventions. There are no short cuts. We are beginning to get better mortality data by age, sex, time, and geography for homicide, but we are only beginning to understand the dimensions of nonfatal outcomes. As Mark Rosenberg points out in the introduction of this book, nonfatal outcomes may represent an even larger social problem than mortality. And we are a long way from knowing how best to use that information to suggest the generic changes most likely to have a favorable impact.

THE CONTEXT OF VIOLENCE

Good national surveillance is one key lesson for us to learn; another is the need to understand violence in its broad context. Most certainly, we should view intentional and unintentional injury together. The surveillance network needs are similar; the risk groups overlap; the risk factors, such as alcohol and depression, overlap; and the instruments, such as cars and guns, overlap. But in addition, violence is not limited to physical injury. Deprivations of many kinds are forms of violence. Discrimination is a form of social violence, as is poverty. Indeed, Gandhi once said that poverty is the worst form of violence. And the threat of nuclear war constitutes a violent cloud over all of us.

Whereas research requires us to narrow the focus, just as we do when studying the nervous system or the gastrointestinal system, this study must be done within a conceptual framework that accommodates the broad scope of violence. It is important to capture the momentum of nonviolent movements and prevent fragmentation of our efforts. The recognition of the International Physicians for the Prevention of Nuclear War for the 1985 Nobel Peace Prize is an important indication that antiviolence movements should be incorporated in the overall strategy.

ROLE OF HEALTH DEPARTMENTS

Health departments should be seen as crucial but not sufficient. This is a lesson learned in many areas, even in what is regarded as standard public health. Health departments are simply not strong enough, sufficiently influential, or rich enough to carry out programs by themselves. Around the world, we see this with immunization programs that become possible only when political leaders and others provide their support. In the United States, polio immunization rates were as low as 65 percent in 1977. It was not until the executive and legislative branches of government became involved with the states and counties, as well as education departments, PTAs, volunteer groups, etc., that immunization rates in this country went to 80 percent, 90 percent, and finally to 97 percent. This comes close to a program of perfection, but it could not have been done by health departments alone.

With violence, it is even more important to involve the largest diversity of professional and volunteer groups possible if a significant impact is to be realized.

What, then, should be the roles of health departments? (1) Health departments could assist to get violence into the mainstream of public health. (2) Health departments could be involved in problem definition, an area of considerable experience and expertise. (3) Health departments could be involved in the education of politicians and those who could change what is now done, education of children through the development of appropriate curricula, and education of the public by providing information to the media. (4) Health departments should develop intervention strategies and evaluate their impact. (5) Health departments must work to keep this interest from being a fad. They must develop the stabilizing interest to sustain a search for answers into the future. This is particularly true if early intervention efforts turn out to be misplaced.

It is important for the federal government to provide leadership, but it is essential that we not wait for the federal government to develop a program. Most health programs at the federal level have evolved because of convincing demonstrations at local levels. This was true for the immunization program, which was built on many private, local, and state demonstrations. One of the telling examples is the use of child restraints in this country. The federal government for a variety of reasons could not or did not provide leadership. A pediatrician and local health officer in Tennessee worked at the county and then the state levels to get the first child restraint law passed in Tennessee. In only a few years, all states had followed the example.

It is important to promote a groundswell of trials, demonstrations, and suggestions from private sources as well as local and state health departments. Many pilot projects of varied types increase the chance of funding some interventions that are worth replicating. You can best force a response from the federal establishment by demonstrating something so compelling that it has to be replicated (as with child restraints).

INTERNATIONAL IMPLICATIONS

Finally, remember the international aspects of violence. There is a great disparity in homicide rates by country and an exceptionally high burden of violence endured by many citizens of the world. Although the developing world is quite correctly concerned with reducing its infectious disease rate, some of these countries are already losing more years of productive life to violence than to infectious diseases. A broad perspective in studying violence and developing intervention strategies will serve the world most completely.

Smallpox is the only disease that has been eliminated from the world. As a person interested in that program, as well as international health generally, I can assure you that you are on the ground floor of something more fundamental and ultimately more important than smallpox eradication. The single most important lesson of smallpox eradication was the demonstration that it is possible to plan a rational health future. What we must do now is a step—a vital step—in planning a rational future for combatting violence.

William Foege, M.D.,
Director, The Carter Center
of Emory University

Contents

Contributors

Ann W. Burgess, R.N., D.N.Sc.
vanAmeringen Professor of
 Psychiatric Mental Health
 Nursing
University of Pennsylvania
Philadelphia, Pennsylvania

David Finkelhor, Ph.D.
Family Violence Research Program
Department of Sociology
University of New Hampshire
Durham, New Hampshire

Anne H. Flitcraft, M.D.
University of Connecticut Health
 Center
Farmington, Connecticut
Co-Director, Domestic Violence
 Training Project
New Haven, Connecticut

William H. Foege, M.D.,
 M.P.H.
Executive Director
The Carter Center of Emory
 University
Atlanta, Georgia

Susan Frankel, Ph.D.
Family Research Laboratory
University of New Hampshire
Durham, New Hampshire

Carol R. Hartman, R.N., D.N.Sc.
Professor of Psychiatric Mental
 Health Nursing
Boston College School of Nursing
Chestnut Hill, Massachusetts

Dean G. Kilpatrick, Ph.D.
Crime Victims Center
Medical University of South Carolina
Charleston, South Carolina

C. Everett Koop, M.D., Sc.D.
Former Surgeon General
U.S. Public Health Service

James A. Mercy, Ph.D.
Division of Injury Control
Center for Environmental Health
 and Injury Control
Centers for Disease Control
Atlanta, Georgia

Eli H. Newberger, M.D.
Children's Hospital
Harvard Medical School
Boston, Massachusetts

Patrick W. O'Carroll, M.D.,
 M.P.H.
Division of Injury Control
Center for Environmental Health
 and Injury Control
Centers for Disease Control
Atlanta, Georgia

Karl Pillemer, Ph.D.
Family Research Laboratory
University of New Hampshire
Durham, New Hampshire

Mark L. Rosenberg, M.D.,
  M.P.P.
Director, Division of Injury
  Control
Center for Environmental Health
  and Injury Control
Centers for Disease Control
Atlanta, Georgia

Evan Stark, Ph.D., M.S.W.
Graduate Department of Public
  Administration
Rutgers University
Newark, New Jersey
Co-Director, Domestic Violence
  Training Project
New Haven, Connecticut

Judith M. Von, Ph.D.
Department of Psychology
University of Virginia
Charlottesville, Virginia

VIOLENCE IN AMERICA

1

Introduction

MARK L. ROSENBERG AND JAMES A. MERCY

VIOLENCE IS A PUBLIC HEALTH PROBLEM

Chances are that on any given day, the daily newspaper of every major U.S. city will present a snapshot of America's growing problem of violence. Articles will cover a range of violent acts: murder, suicide, assault, child abuse, and rape. Although these daily stories catch people's attention, readers all too often view the violence as a fact of life, something that is unpredictable and unpreventable. Our society and even health and public health professionals too infrequently realize that violence is a problem that can be studied, understood, and prevented (1).

There were over 20,000 homicides and 31,000 suicides in this country in 1987, and nonfatal assaults and suicide attempts may outnumber homicides and suicides by a ratio of more than 100 to 1 (2–4). Assaults include incidents ranging from sexual assault, robbery, and gang warfare to domestic violence. Although there is some controversy over the actual numbers and rates for the incidence of rape as well as the extent of underreporting, the Federal Bureau of Investigation considers rape a serious crime, second only to murder. Increases in the rate of rape (21%) were the greatest among all major crimes from 1977 to 1984 (5). Estimates of the prevalence of spouse abuse indicate that approximately 20 percent of adult women in the United States have been physically abused at least once by a male intimate. In 1986 according to the annual 50-state survey of the National Committee for Prevention of Child Abuse, an estimated two million reports of child abuse and neglect were filed (6), representing a 6 percent increase over the previous year.

For every statistic cited, there is a face. Indeed, for all types of violence except suicide, there are at least two faces: a victim and a perpetrator. Many faces are young—children who are physically or sexually abused and growing numbers of youth who commit suicide. In 1950 the suicide rate for persons 15–24 years of age was 4.5 per 100,000; in 1988 this rate was 12.8 (4). Other faces are disproportionately young and black. The homicide rates for young black men are five times as high as the rates for white men in the same age group, and homicide rates for black women are higher than those for white men. The lifetime probability of becoming a homicide victim among babies born in the United States in 1989 ranged from 1:496 for a white female baby to 1:27 for a black male baby (7). Other characteristics associated with victims and perpetrators, particularly for homicide and assault, include alcohol and drug use, low socioeconomic status, and the availability of firearms.

The traditional public policy response to interpersonal violence has assigned responsibility to the criminal justice system and has focused prevention on deterrence and incapacitation. However, rates for all violent crimes have increased, suggesting that this approach is not adequate. In the years since World War II, Americans concerned about health and well-being have seen a shift in the impact of violence at the same time they saw a decrease in the impact of communicable diseases. During the early postwar years, vaccines and therapeutic treatments were developed that protected people against diseases that had caused a good deal of death and disability in our society. In the same years, death and disability from interpersonal violence began to increase. We can and will find ways to protect ourselves from the threat of violence, but we need to look beyond the biomedical armamentarium of "magic bullets."

The traditional approach to suicide prevention has also been narrowly focused not on criminal justice, but on the mental health sector. Suicide was considered a problem that psychologists and psychiatrists could take care of. They were taught that suicide was a problem for depressed, older white men, and if they identified these older white men at risk, they could treat their depression and thereby prevent suicide. Yet beginning in 1980, for the first time, most persons who committed suicide in the United States were 40 years of age or younger. And among young men, ages 15–24, where the suicide rates more than tripled between 1950 and 1980, the people committing suicide were generally not depressed. Instead they were impulsive and likely to have been in trouble at home, in school, and with the police. They were unlikely to walk into a psychiatrist's or psychologist's office and certainly did not fit the traditional profile of the person at risk. Thus as with homicide, to address suicide prevention effectively, we need to look beyond the traditional approaches, beyond the domain of mental health clinicians.

One way to measure the cost of violence is through the morbidity and mortality associated with it. Suicide is the eighth leading cause of death, and homicide ranks twelfth (9). However, ranking health problems by their overall status as a cause of death does not take into account the age at which people die from that problem. Another measure of the public health importance of a problem would be an indicator of the potential years of life lost because of that particular problem. For example, if age 65 is the average length of a productive life, then a death at age 64 would result in the loss of one year of productive life; a death at age 20 would result in the loss of 45 years of potential productive life. When calculated in terms of potential life lost (YPLL), homicide ranked fourth and suicide, fifth in 1984 (9).

Although the data on nonfatal outcomes of violence are scarce and inadequate, there is overwhelming evidence that morbidity associated with violence represents a tremendous cost to society and the victims. Throughout the chapters of this book, these outcomes, which include physical and psychological injuries, are described for each type of violence. In order to place psychological injury into proper perspective, much more information is needed concerning the victim's subsequent problems with drug and alcohol abuse, increased rates of suicide, and other forms of self-destructive behavior, including overly aggressive or violent behavior as well as passive behavior that puts them at risk of further victimization. The economic costs of violence include the cost of medical care and psychological counseling for victims, the cost of legal proceedings and incarceration of perpetrators, and the loss in earnings of those who die or who are incapacitated by a violent act. The economic cost to the nation of all injuries incurred in 1988 was estimated to be $180 billion (10). If these costs follow the pattern of injury fatalities—where one third of all injury deaths are from intentional injury or violence—then the cost of violent injuries may be about $60 billion annually. These costs, it should be noted, do not include the psychological suffering and disruption attenuated upon families whose members sustain intentional injuries nor the pain and suffering of the victims themselves.

FIREARM INJURIES: A PUBLIC HEALTH PRIORITY

During 1986 and 1987, the number of people who died from firearm injuries in the United States (66,182) was greater than the number of casualties suffered during the entire eight and one-half years of conflict in Vietnam. Gunshot wounds are the second leading cause of injury mortality, ranking behind motor vehicle crashes. In 1987, 32,857 persons died as a result of firearm injuries. Over 90 percent of these fatalities were due to suicide and homicide. Firearm mortality rates for women, male teenagers, and young adults have been higher during the 1980s than at any time previously.

Nonfatal firearm injuries often result in major disabilities. In Detroit, 40 percent of all traumatic spinal cord injury results from gunshot wounds. In 1985 firearm injuries imposed a $14.4 billion economic burden on the United States (9). The health and economic burden imposed by firearm injuries is much higher in the United States than for other industrialized countries. For example, homicide rates for men 15–24 years of age in Israel, Canada, Japan, West Germany, and other industrialized countries are all less than one-fifth the equivalent rate in the United States.

The public health community must help to promote and establish a more complete scientific understanding of the role of firearms in homicide, suicide, and unintentional injury (11). Major advances in the prevention of public health problems, such as motor vehicle injuries, have been achieved through the application of sound scientific principles. Applying these principles will allow the development of an information base necessary for identifying effective strategies for preventing firearm injuries. Research findings need to be disseminated so that citizens, policymakers, and others can make informed judgments on how to prevent firearm injuries. This must be done in a way that allows flexibility for states and localities to define which mix of outcomes and strategies will best achieve the goal of preventing firearm injuries, given their particular resources and political environment.

There are three major scientific priorities that must be addressed to establish a solid foundation for the prevention of firearm injuries:

1. The magnitude and distribution of firearm-related morbidity, disability, and behavioral risk factors should be routinely monitored through public health surveillance systems.
2. High priority should be given to epidemiologic investigations that focus on quantifying the risks for injury associated with firearm possession or lack thereof in individuals.
3. Regulations and other interventions that potentially affect the risk of firearm injury must be rigorously evaluated.

Little is known about the magnitude and distribution of firearm-related morbidity and disability. More complete and accurate measurement of the incidence, prevalence, and costs of firearm injury would help to establish the priority that should be given to their health consequences. In addition, we lack routinely collected information on behavioral risk factors (e.g., gun storage and accessibility to loaded weapons) that contribute to firearm-associated morbidity and mortality. Information on these factors would help to establish the characteristics of persons with easy access to guns so that high-risk groups could be targeted for intervention. In addition, such information would help evaluate efforts aimed at preventing firearm injury, reducing access, and altering unsafe storage practices.

YEAR 2000 OBJECTIVES SET PRIORITIES

Faced with the overwhelming burden of premature death and disability caused by violence and confident of the ability of epidemiological methods to help with the problem, the public health community made intentional injury a priority in the public health agenda in the early 1980s. One of the first public acknowledgements of the inclusion of intentional injury as a public health problem came with the 1979 publication of *Promoting Health/Preventing Disease: Objectives for the Nation*. Objectives addressing homicide, child abuse, and suicide were included in those specific health objectives for the nation targeted to be achieved by 1990. In the 1980s the

Centers for Disease Control became the lead agency for coordination of injury control activities. The CDC program provided support for injury prevention research grants in seven universities; administered 70 grants awarded to state and local governments, universities and community organizations; and conducted intramural research. In assessing the CDC program impact, the National Academy of Sciences in 1988 published an evaluation report, *Injury Control* (12), which stated that the "value of the program has been established beyond expectation: researchers have suggested innovative projects far in excess of research resources; educators have introduced new courses in graduate schools; public health programs have sprung to life in state and local health departments across the country; and morbidity and mortality rates are beginning to decline for many categories of injury."

As America approaches the millennium, the Public Health Service is evaluating the success of the health objectives set for 1990 and is setting objectives to be reached by the year 2000 (13). The increase in the number and scope of health objectives that relate to intentional injury in the Year 2000 Health Objectives reflects the growing importance and more aggressive efforts in this area. Baseline data for the Year 2000 Objectives, where available, are from 1985, 1986, and 1987. Throughout this book, statistics are from the same years, which is the latest information available and analyzed.

The Year 2000 Health Objectives for Violent and Abusive Behavior are divided into objectives for health status, risk reduction, and services and protection (13).

Health Status Objectives

Reduce Homicides to No More than 7.2 per 100,000 People (Rate in 1987 = 8.5 per 100,000)

Writers of the objectives cited that men, teenagers, young adults, and minority group members, particularly blacks and Hispanics, are consistently found to be at greatest risk of homicide victimization; that poverty is an extremely important risk factor for homicide; and that the use, manufacture, and distribution of drugs are also important factors influencing the risk of homicide.

Reduce Suicides to No More than 10.5 per 100,000 People (Rate in 1987 = 11.7 per 100,000)

Suicide rates are highest among white men and Native Americans and the major method of committing suicide in the United States is by firearm. Rates for all youth, ages 15–19, have been increasing since the 1950s; in 1986 suicide was the second leading cause of death among people of this age group. Suicide rates for men, ages 20–34, have increased dramatically in the last three decades and have remained high since 1978 (25.0/100,000). Rates are highest for persons age 65 and older.

Reduce Weapon-Related Violent Deaths to No More than 12.6 per 100,000 People
(Rate in 1987 = 12.9 per 100,000 [by Firearms])

Firearms rank second, after motor vehicles, as the greatest contributor to injury mortality. Firearm suicides and homicides account for over 90 percent of all firearm related deaths. Of all suicides and homicides that occur in the United States, about 60 percent are attributed to firearms.

Reverse to Less than 25.2 per 1,000 Children the Rising Incidence of Maltreatment of Children Under Age 18
(Rate in 1986 = 25.2 per 1,000)

Child maltreatment is defined in federal legislation as the physical or mental injury, sexual abuse or exploitation, negligent treatment, or maltreatment of a child by a person who is responsible for the child's welfare under circumstances that indicate the child's health or welfare is harmed or threatened. There are difficulties with valid and reliable measurements of child maltreatment. National data collected usually only reflect incidents known to child protection agencies, other investigatory agencies, or professionals in schools, hospitals, and other major agencies. It is not possible to determine whether trends in these data sources reflect increases in the reporting and identification of maltreatment or increases in the magnitude of child maltreatment in the United States.

Reduce Rape and Attempted Rape of Women Age 12 and Older to No More than 107 per 100,000 Women
(Rate in 1986 = 120 per 100,000)

Self-report data from the National Crime Survey on rape and attempted rape indicate that young, unmarried, and low-income women are at highest risk. Women between the ages of 12 and 34 are at particularly high risk. The rates of attempted and completed rape are difficult to measure accurately because many victims do not report or discuss the experience, particularly victims of acquaintance rape or date rape.

Reduce Physical Abuse Directed at Women by Male Partners to No More than 27 per 1,000 Couples
(Rate in 1985 = 30 per 1,000 Couples)

Women are more at risk for assault and rape by a male partner than by a stranger. Additionally, women are often battered by their partners during pregnancy. The baseline rate for this objective estimates severe violence, defined as acts that have a relatively high probability of causing an injury.

Reduce Assault Injuries among People Age 12 and Older to No More than 10 per 1,000 People (Rate in 1986 = 11.1 per 1,000)

An assault injury is defined as any physical or bodily harm occurring during the course of a rape, robbery, or any other type of attack upon a person. An estimated 28 percent of violent crime victims suffered injuries; over 13 percent had injuries serious enough to require medical attention; 7 percent of injuries were serious enough to require hospital care; and for 1 percent, a hospital stay was necessary. Rates of injury from violent and abusive behavior were highest for males, blacks, people ages 19–24, people who were separated or divorced, those earning less than $10,000 per year, and residents of central cities.

Reduce by 15 Percent the Incidence of Injurious Suicide Attempts among Adolescents Aged 14 through 19 (Baseline Unavailable)

Attempted suicide is a morbid, potentially lethal health event and a risk factor for future completed suicide. It is also a potential indicator of other health problems such as substance abuse, depression, or adjustment or stress reactions.

Risk Reduction Objectives

Reduce by 20 Percent the Incidence of Physical Fighting among Adolescents Ages 14 to 17 (Baseline to be Established in 1991)

Physical fighting among adolescents is often considered a normal and sometimes necessary part of growing up. Physical fighting, however, results in hundreds of homicides and uncounted numbers of nonfatal injuries among adolescents each year. In many instances of homicide and serious assaultive injury, physical fighting may be considered a necessary, if not a sufficient, cause for the death or injury. A reduction in the incidence of physical fighting may prove extremely important in disrupting the causal mechanisms of homicide and assaultive injury.

Reduce by 20 Percent the Incidence of Weapon-Carrying by Adolescents Ages 14 through 17 (Baseline to be Established in 1991)

Approximately six out of ten homicide victims in the United States are killed with firearms; nine out of ten are killed with a weapon of some type, such as a gun, knife, or club. Although the question of restricting firearm ownership and usage is a contentious one in American society, few argue that adolescents should have unsupervised access to firearms or other lethal weapons. This objective seeks to reduce and monitor this high-risk behavior.

Reduce by 20 Percent the Proportion of Weapons that Are Inappropriately Stored and Thereby Dangerously Available (Baseline to be Established in 1991)

Because of the lethal nature of firearms and the impulsive nature of many homicides, it is possible that many homicides and suicides could be prevented if immediate access to firearms was reduced. There are a broad range of environmental and behavioral measures that may be effective in reducing the immediate access of certain sectors of the population to loaded firearms (e.g., placing weapons in locked places so that children have no access to them and restricting the legality of carrying loaded firearms in public).

Services and Protection Objectives

Extend Protocols for Routinely Identifying, Treating, and Properly Referring Suicide Attempts, Victims of Sexual Assault, and Victims of Spouse, Elder, and Child Abuse to at Least 90 Percent of Hospital Emergency Departments (Baseline Data Unavailable)

Efforts by hospital emergency departments to adopt standard protocols to facilitate and make routine the early recognition of such victims and timely referral for appropriate intervention and treatment can lower the death and injury rate due to violent or abusive behavior including the emotional consequences associated with repeated exposure.

Extend to at Least Forty-Five States Implementation of Unexplained Child Death Review Systems (Baseline Data Unavailable)

State-of-the-art practices in child death investigation are important for accurately identifying child abuse deaths, assuring that living children in families in which child abuse deaths occur are adequately protected, and determining how child abuse death cases could have been managed more effectively by agencies with which the child victims had contact.

Increase to at Least Thirty the Number of States in Which at Least 50 Percent of Children Identified as Physically or Sexually Abused Receive Physical and Mental Evaluation with Appropriate Followup as a Means of Breaking the Intergenerational Cycle of Abuse (Baseline Data Unavailable)

Standard diagnostic protocols are needed to detect the abused child's devalued self-image, loss of trust, and distorted view of parent-child relationships in order to prevent the tendency for abused children to perpetuate the abusive relationship they have with their parents in subsequent relationships. The results of these assessments should be used to provide these children with appropriate therapeutic treatments.

Reduce to Less than 10 Percent the Proportion of Battered Women and their Children Turned Away from Emergency Housing due to the Lack of Space (Baseline in 1987 = 40%)

The lack of available space for battered women and their children could be partially alleviated if more shelters for battered women and their children were available. Also, if more nonresidential programs were available, some women might consider various options earlier in the battering cycle, thus avoiding severe battering and the need for shelter services.

Increase to at Least 50 Percent the Proportion of Elementary and Secondary Schools that Teach Nonviolent Conflict Resolution Skills, Preferably as a Part of Quality School Health Education (Baseline Data not Available)

Conflict resolution and violence prevention curricula have been developed for various grade levels. Although studies of the effectiveness of these curricula in reducing violent and abusive behaviors are inconclusive, these curricula seem promising.

Extend Coordinated, Comprehensive Violence Prevention Programs to at Least 80 Percent of States and Local Jurisdictions with Populations over 100,000 (Baseline Data Unavailable)

A coordinated, comprehensive effort by state and local health, criminal justice, and social service agencies is necessary to maximize resources and ensure the availability of violence prevention strategies and information to all segments of the population. Collaboration across these traditionally disparate agencies is necessary in order to break down barriers that impede the advancement of violence prevention and control activities.

Increase to 50 the Number of States with Officially Established Protocols that Engage Mental Health, Alcohol and Drug, and Public Health Authorities with Corrections Authorities to Facilitate Identification and Appropriate Intervention to Prevent Suicide by Jail Inmates (Baseline Data Unavailable)

Suicide is the leading cause of death in U.S. jails. The suicide rate among inmates in county jails and police lockups is 16 times greater than that for individuals in the general population. Only 36 of the 50 states have either voluntary or mandatory jail standards regarding suicide. Only 8 state jail standards specify inquiry concerning suicidal behavior in their intake screening, and fewer than 12 state jail standards have specific policies and procedures regarding the prevention of suicide. Two states specify continuous observation for certain groups of suicidal inmates.

AN INTERDISCIPLINARY APPROACH TO VIOLENCE

Solving the problem of violence will require an interdisciplinary approach. Professionals from sociology, criminology, economics, law, public policy, psychology, anthropology, and public health must work together to understand the causes and develop the solutions. Neither causes nor solutions will be simple. To collaborate effectively, these disciplines must agree upon definitions and build compatible data sets. Programs need to be shared, building new bridges with service delivery institutions that are traditionally outside the venue of health agencies, including community-based services like shelters for battered women and rape crisis centers.

The contribution of public health to this arena has been to bring to society's attention the recognition that violence is a public health problem, and then to apply epidemiologic techniques, the use of surveillance systems and other data collection systems, and the development and implementation of preventive strategies (14). The public health approach has begun to identify underlying patterns of violence that will help us understand who is at high risk and what risk factors are associated with particular types of violence (15).

Public health also addresses the social norms and attitudes that accept violence as a part of American life. The perception that violence is inevitable is unacceptable to those who work to improve our nation's health and quality of life. We believe that violence is a difficult problem, a multifaceted problem, but one that can be characterized, analyzed, and effectively controlled by understanding and action. If this understanding and action come from all these disciplines that come into contact with the thousands of victims of violence in the United States, we can and will make a significant difference.

REFERENCES

1. Rosenberg ML. Violence is a public health problem. In: Maulitz RC, ed. Unnatural Causes: The three leading killer diseases in America. New Brunswick, NJ: Rutgers University Press, 1989.
2. Rosenberg ML, Mercy J. Homicide: Epidemiologic analysis at the national level. Bull NY Acad Med 1986; 62(5):376–394.
3. US Dept of Justice, Bureau of Justice Statistics. Criminal victimization in the United States, 1986: A National Crime Survey report. Washington, DC: Bureau of Justice Statistics, US Dept. of Justice (NCJ-111456), 1988.
4. National Center for Health Statistics. Advance report of final mortality statistics, 1987. Hyattsville, MD: National Center for Health Statistics. DHHS pub no (PHS)89-1120 (Monthly Vital Statistics Report; vol 38, no 5 suppl).
5. US Dept of Justice, Federal Bureau of Investigation. Crime in the United States: Uniform crime reports. Washington, DC: US Govt Printing Office, 1982.
6. Daro D, Mitchel L. Deaths due to maltreatment soar: The results of the 1986 annual fifty state survey. Chicago: National Center on Child Abuse Prevention Research, National Committee for Prevention of Child Abuse, 1987.
7. Federal Bureau of Investigation. Uniform crime reports, 1989. Washington, DC: US Dept. of Justice, 1990.
8. Shaffer D. Strategies for prevention of youth suicide. Publ Health Rep 1987; 102(6):611–614.
9. Centers for Disease Control. Premature mortality due to suicide and homicide— United States, 1984: Perspectives in disease prevention and health promotion. MMWR August 21, 1987; 36(32):531–534.
10. Rice DP, MacKenzie EJ, et al. Cost of injury in the United States: A report to Congress. San Francisco: Institute for Health and Aging, University of California and Injury Prevention Center, Johns Hopkins University, 1989.

11. Mercy JA, Houk VN. Firearm injuries: A call for science. N Engl J Med 1988; 319(19):1283–1285.
12. National Academy of Sciences. Injury control: A review of the status and progress of the Injury Control Program at the Centers for Disease Control. Washington, D.C.: National Academy Press, 1988.
13. Public Health Service: Year 2000 Health Objectives. Washington, DC: US Govt. Printing Office, 1990.
14. The National Committee for Injury Prevention and Control. Injury prevention: Meeting the challenge. New York: Oxford University Press, 1989.
15. Mercy JA, O'Carroll PW. New directions in violence prediction: The public health arena. Violence and Victims 1988; 3(4):285–301.

2

Assaultive Violence

MARK L. ROSENBERG AND JAMES A. MERCY

Assaultive violence is a very serious public health problem in the United States, with consequences of psychological and social dysfunction as well as injury and death. Assaultive violence includes both nonfatal and fatal interpersonal violence where physical force or other means is used by one person with the intent of causing harm, injury, or death to another. Homicide is death due to injuries inflicted by another person with intent to harm, injure, or kill by any means. In 1986 homicide was the twelfth leading cause of death overall in the United States and the leading cause of death for black men aged 15–34. In addition, in the United States, homicide was the fourth leading cause of potential years of life lost—an index that measures the number of years of productive life lost to society through the deaths of persons who died before reaching age 65. This highlights the important impact of this problem on our nation's youth.

Nonfatal assaults may constitute an even more important aspect of this public health problem than homicide. The estimated magnitude of this problem is smaller if based upon crimes reported to the police; larger if based upon self-reported incidents. In 1985 the ratio of nonfatal assaultive crimes (reported to police) to homicides was about 69:1. Estimates of the number of completed nonfatal violent assaults based on self-reports (i.e., those reported in the National Crime Survey) to homicides exceeds 100:1, and these figures may still underestimate the true extent of nonfatal assaultive violence in the United States.

Data on assaultive violence are available at the national, state, and local levels from both criminal justice and health sources. Nationally, the Federal Bureau of Investigation (FBI) through the Uniform Crime Reporting System (UCR) compiles data on all crimes known to police for each year in addition to collecting more detailed information on homicides, including information about the victim/offender relationship and circumstances of the homicide. The National Center for Health Statistics (NCHS) compiles information on homicide based on death certificates received from the 50 states and the District of Columbia. Criminal justice sources for data on nonfatal assaultive violence include the National Crime Survey conducted by the Bureau of Justice Statistics and UCR data compiled by the FBI. Potentially useful health sources for nonfatal assaultive violence include the National Health Interview Survey, the National Hospital Discharge Survey, and the National Electronic Injury Surveillance System. State and local level data on assaultive violence are available from criminal justice agencies, hospitals through discharge information and admissions to emergency rooms, medical examiners' and coroners' offices, and a variety of social service agencies.

Data needs are much greater for nonfatal assaults than for homicide. There is an urgent need for better data on injuries resulting from nonfatal assaults and for surveillance of nonfatal assaultive violence at the state and local levels.

Assaultive violence is a common endpoint of many quite different behavioral pathways, such as arguments between acquaintances, escalating domestic violence between spouses, or robberies perpetrated by strangers. Each pathway or type of assaultive violence may be associated with a unique set of causes and risk factors. Current thinking on the causes of assaultive violence suggests that biological factors (such as male sex, young age, or mental illness), psychological factors (such as history of previous abuse, history of violent behavior by parents), cultural factors (such as male belief in physical prowess and media glorification of violence), "structural" or large-scale social factors (such as poverty and racial discrimination), and interactionist factors (such as alcohol and drug abuse) all may contribute to assaultive violence. There is a need to develop theoretical perspectives that take into account this multidimensional nature of assaultive violence and that clarify those situations and circumstances that can promote or prevent assaultive violence.

Assaultive violence causes 19,000 to 23,000 deaths each year in the United States, taking its greatest toll among minorities, men, and the young. Young black men have experienced homicide rates five to ten times higher than those for young white men during the last two decades. Young Hispanic men and black women also have disproportionately high homicide rates. Almost half of all homicides occur among persons who know one another; in two-thirds of these instances the perpetrator and victim are friends or acquaintances; in one-third, they are family members. Firearms are the weapons used in approximately 60 percent of all homicides. Based on the National Crime Survey, there have been over two million completed nonfatal violent crimes each year since 1980 among persons age 12 and over in the United States in addition to over 3.5 million attempted violent crimes. As with homicide, minorities, men, and the young are at greatest risk.

Little is known about how to prevent interpersonal violence most effectively. However, strategies to prevent assaultive violence should include efforts to induce broad social changes while simultaneously promoting the implementation of specific interventions by various public sectors. Social and cultural changes include efforts to decrease the cultural acceptance of violence, reduce racial discrimination, reduce gender inequality, and support more flexible male role models. The health and related social services sector should evaluate the potential costs and benefits of a variety of intervention strategies. Potential strategies include:

1. Developing and implementing educational programs to teach conflict-resolution skills.
2. Increasing and enriching educational programs for family life, family planning, and child-rearing.
3. Developing sources of family support through community-based support services.
4. Improving the identification of victims of violence in health-care and social-service settings.
5. Providing incentives for health-care personnel to become involved in cases of violence.
6. Improving the management and treatment of victims of violence.
7. Improving the ability of the health-care system to recognize and treat the social and psychological consequences of violence as well as the physical injuries.
8. Decreasing the financial barriers to care for victims.
9. Improving the identification and treatment of perpetrators of violence by our health-care and social-service systems.
10. Improving record-keeping and reporting for victims of assaultive violence.
11. Improving communication and cooperation among health-care providers, police departments, social service agencies, and schools.

Similarly, there are a number of strategies that deserve evaluation by the criminal justice sector, including:

1. Directing police to treat physical assaults among persons who know each other (e.g., family, intimates, and acquaintances) as criminal behavior.
2. Training police and citizen intervention teams.
3. Coordinating the responses of police and social services to assaultive violence.
4. Initiating informal citizen surveillance and silent witness programs.
5. Facilitating the access of victims to legal services.
6. Initiating victim- and witness-assistance programs.
7. Developing programs to train high-risk adolescents and providing job opportunities for them.
8. Focusing on prevention in the treatment of illness related to the consumption of alcohol and other drugs.

STATEMENT OF THE PROBLEM

Overview

Assaultive violence is now clearly recognized as an important public health problem. Each year, over 20,000 people die from homicide in the United States, making it the twelfth leading cause of death and the fourth leading cause of premature mortality (1). Whereas homicide represents the most serious outcome, assaultive behaviors are many times more common than homicide and are very diverse in their characteristics (e.g., sexual assault, robbery, gang warfare, domestic arguments). The ratio of nonfatal assaults to homicide is probably far greater than 100:1 (2).

Violence has particularly serious health implications for young people in this country. Among those 15–24 years of age, homicide ranks as the third leading cause of death. Even more striking is the fact that homicide is the leading cause of death for black men 15–34 years of age and that the lifetime risk of death from homicide is one in 28 for black men compared with one in 164 for white men (3,4).

In the past, assaultive violence has been considered the concern of the criminal justice system alone, and control strategies have relied almost exclusively on the capabilities and resources of law enforcement, judicial, and penal institutions. These strategies, focused primarily on deterrence through punishment and imprisonment, have not succeeded in reducing homicide rates or rates of nonfatal assaults. In fact, the past 30 years have witnessed dramatic increases in homicide rates in the United States: in 1980, the homicide rate reached its highest recorded level of the century (5). Defining homicide as a public health problem suggests that it is a concern to be addressed and remedied, not an inalterable fact of life. We believe that public health with its focus on epidemiologic analysis and prevention can make a substantial contribution to reducing the enormous toll in deaths and injuries attributable to assaultive violence in this country.

This chapter presents an assessment of assaultive violence in the United States as a public health problem. The public health approach has come to represent, through repeated application and refinement, a unified framework for developing relevant information and transferring that information into effective action. The science through which information is analyzed to enhance the prevention of public health problems is epidemiology, or the study of the occurrence and distribution of disease and other health-related conditions in human populations (6). The epidemiologic approach to the development of information can be summarized in four interrelated steps: (1) *public health surveillance*, i.e., the development and refinement of data systems for the ongoing and systematic collection, analysis, interpretation, and dissemination of health data; (2) *risk group identification*, i.e., the identification of persons at greatest risk of disease or injury and the places, times, and other circumstances that are associated with increased risk; (3) *risk factor identification*, i.e., the analytic exploration of potentially causative risk factors for disease or death as suggested by the nature of the high-risk population and other research; and (4) *program development, implementation, and evaluation*, i.e., the design, implementation, and evaluation of preventive interventions based on our understanding of the population at risk and the risk factors for the outcome of interest (7).

Definitions

In this chapter we use the term *assaultive violence* to include both nonfatal and fatal interpersonal violence where physical force by one person is used with the intent of causing harm, injury, or death to another. *Homicide* is death due to injuries inflicted through any means by another person with intent to injure or kill. Homicide may be further classified as either criminal or noncriminal. Criminal homicide excludes death caused by negligence and justifiable homicides (i.e., those committed in self-defense or in the line of duty by a police officer).

Four legal categories are commonly used to identify nonfatal assaultive violence in surveillance, research, and media reports: aggravated assault, simple assault, rape, and robbery. *Aggravated assault* is defined as either (1) an attack with a weapon, whether or not there is injury; (2) an attack without a weapon resulting either in serious injury (e.g., broken bones, loss of teeth, internal injuries, loss of consciousness) or in undetermined injury requiring two or more days of hospitalization; or (3) an attempted assault with a weapon (2). It is important to remember that, as legally defined, aggravated assault represents only one category of assault. Thus to be included in the category of aggravated assault as used in most existing data sets, an event must fit a fairly narrow definition that may not be the most useful for public health purposes. Aggravated assault should also be distinguished from simple assault. *Simple assault* is defined as an attack (or attempted attack) without a weapon resulting either in minor injury (e.g., bruises, black eyes, cuts, scratches, or swelling) or in undetermined injury requiring less than two days of hospitalization (2). Research literature generally presents assault and homicide as similar categories of behavior and considers homicide as a "completed" assault. Consequently, most strategies that would reduce assault are also generally presumed to reduce homicides. *Rape* is carnal knowledge through the use of force or the threat of force, including attempts (2). *Robbery* is a completed or attempted theft directly from a person of property or cash by force or threat of force, with or without a weapon (2).

Assaultive violence, both fatal and nonfatal, can be divided into different types based on characteristics such as victim-offender relationship, setting, and circumstance. The most commonly used means of categorizing assaultive violence is by the nature of the victim-offender relationship. This approach is useful because both the etiology and prevention strategies for assaultive violence vary by the victim-offender relationship. In this chapter we distinguish between three general categories of assaultive violence: family, acquaintance, and stranger.

DATA SOURCES

A variety of routinely collected sources of data on assaultive violence exist at
the national, state, and local levels in the United States. However, important
gaps in the quality and availability of information remain despite the variety
of data sources available, particularly with respect to nonfatal assaultive
violence. In this section we describe sources of available data on assaultive
violence and review their strengths and limitations.

National Data Sources

Federal Bureau of Investigation (FBI)
Uniform Crime Reports (UCR)
The FBI-UCR program receives information monthly from over 16,000
city, county, and state law enforcement agencies. This is a voluntary program intended to generate reliable criminal statistics for use in law enforcement administration. During 1986 the law enforcement agencies in the UCR
program held jurisdiction over 96 percent of the U.S. population (8). These
law enforcement agencies report the number of "actual offenses known" for
murder and nonnegligent manslaughter (i.e., criminal homicide), justifiable
homicide, negligent manslaughter, forcible rape, robbery, aggravated assault, burglary, larceny-theft, motor vehicle theft, and arson.

For all reported homicides, the FBI-UCR program uses a Supplementary
Homicide Report (SHR) to collect information on the age, race, and sex of
the victim and offender; the relationship of the offender to the victim; and
information on the crime circumstances. These reports are completed and
forwarded to the FBI from local, county, and state law enforcement agencies at the end of each month. For cases that are unsolved at the time of
reporting, the relationship between offender and victim is listed as unknown. Although this relationship may subsequently be clarified by the
reporting agency, the initial report (relationship unknown), unless specifically amended, stands and is counted in the final statistics for the year. Each
year, data are incomplete for approximately 5–10 percent of the total
murder and nonnegligent manslaughter cases because either (1) the reporting agencies do not submit SHRs for cases initially listed on the summary
report of actual offenses known, or (2) the agencies do not submit reports to
the UCR program for all or part of the year.

FBI-UCR data on aggravated assault, robbery, and rape present several
limitations to epidemiologic research and surveillance. First, these data
represent only those violent offenses known to the police. The majority of
nonfatal violent offenses, in fact, do not come to the attention of law
enforcement agencies. In a study of injuries treated in emergency rooms in
the Cleveland and Lorain-Elyria Standard Metropolitan Statistical Areas
(SMSA), Barancik et al. found that approximately four times more cases of
nonfatal assaultive violence come to the attention of hospitals than to local
police (9). Second, the FBI-UCR program does not collect information on

victim and offender characteristics or relationships for aggravated assaults, robberies, or rapes. Third, the FBI-UCR data on assault are affected by the crime hierarchy that this system uses. If a criminal incident includes several different acts, only the most "serious" act is counted. The UCR ranks homicide as most serious, followed by rape, robbery, aggravated assault, burglary, larceny, and motor vehicle theft. Thus a person who was robbed and assaulted would be classified as a robbery victim, and the incident would be classified as a robbery in the UCR.

A summary of the data collected through this program is published annually in *Crime in the United States* (8). More detailed discussions of the strengths and limitations of this data source can be found elsewhere (10–17). Plans for significant revisions in the FBI-UCR program are currently being formulated. Contemplated changes for the FBI-UCR include collecting more detailed data on victim/offender characteristics in crimes other than homicide and eliminating the crime hierarchy.

National Crime Survey (NCS)

In the literature on assaultive violence, many estimates of the impact of violence are based on the U.S. Department of Justice's annual National Crime Survey (NCS). The NCS was developed by the Bureau of Justice Statistics (BJS) of the U.S. Department of Justice to provide detailed information about the victims and consequences of crime, to estimate the numbers and types of crimes not reported to police, and to establish uniform measures for selected types of crimes in order to permit reliable comparisons over time and between areas (18). These surveys focus on personal and household victimization for six selected crimes: rape, robbery, assault, burglary, larceny, and motor vehicle theft. In 1986 approximately 100,000 individuals age 12 and over, inhabiting approximately 49,000 housing units, participated in the survey (2). All persons age 12 or over within each selected housing unit were eligible to be interviewed, and information on each personal and household victimization was recorded. The data collected include information on physical injury, medical treatment, property loss, characteristics of the victim, relationship of the victim to the offender, and whether or not the police were notified.

This survey is an excellent source of information about victimization and its consequences because it is based upon interviews with victims and is not dependent on official law enforcement records. The National Crime Survey, however, has several limitations that may contribute to the undercounting of assaultive violence. First, the accuracy of this survey's information on injuries and victimizations due to crimes such as spouse, child, and elder abuse is questionable since interviews with household members are not conducted privately and subjects may be reluctant to provide information about family victims or to speak openly in the presence of persons who have victimized them. Moreover, the survey solicits information about criminal assaults, and respondents may not perceive and report assaults by family members as criminal assaults. Second, those groups at highest risk for serious injury from assault may be the most difficult to reach using the household sampling and interviewing techniques applied in the survey. Third, estimates derived from this survey employ the crime hierarchy system used in the FBI-UCR, so that the more serious crimes will be more accurately estimated than crimes lower in the hierarchy. Findings of this survey are published in annual summaries entitled *Criminal Victimization in the United States* (2) and in periodic reports on particular subjects by the BJS.

National Center for Health Statistics (NCHS) Mortality Data

The Vital Statistics of NCHS has collected records of all deaths in the United States from death certificates filed in state vital statistics offices since 1933. This system produces annual data on homicide for the nation and for individual states, counties, and other local areas and monthly provisional data for the nation and each state. The findings are published in the *Monthly Vital Statistics Report*, the annual *Vital Statistics of the United States*, and Series 20 and 21 of the *Vital and Health Statistics Series*. Rates and numbers, gender, and geographic detail for all deaths are published monthly (19), but there is considerable delay in the publication of detailed reports on specific causes of death such as homicide.

Data are collected based on the International Classification of Diseases (ICD) codes (20). The Supplementary External Cause (E) code for homicide includes deaths from injuries purposely inflicted by other persons (ICD-9, codes E960-E969), deaths from injuries resulting from intervention by law enforcement officers (ICD-9, codes E970-E977), and deaths caused by legal execution (ICD-9, code E978).

The current coding system for homicide has limitations. For example, the E-codes and the death certificate information for homicide do not include such essential information as the victim-offender relationship, nor do they permit the distinction between criminal homicides and homicides perpetrated in self-defense.

Other Potentially Useful National Data Sources

Three other national data sources are potentially useful for conducting surveillance and research on assaultive violence if substantial modifications are made in the types of information collected. These data sources include the National Health Interview Survey (NHIS), National Hospital Discharge Survey (NHDS), and National Electronic Injury Surveillance System (NEISS).

The NHIS collects data on the prevalence of chronic diseases and impairments, disability, illness, injury, physician and dental visits, and other health topics. The reports are based on interviews conducted in about 42,000 households sampled to be representative of the civilian, noninstitutionalized population. Conducted annually since 1957, the NHIS is published in Series 10 of the Vital and Health Statistics Series. Currently, however, the information asked about injuries cannot be broken down by the cause of the injury (e.g., assaultive violence, suicidal behavior, unintentional injury). In addition, there is considerable ambiguity in the way questions are asked. For example, it is often unclear as to whether they are asking about all injuries, regardless of intent, or just about unintentional injuries. These limitations must be remedied before this database will be useful for studying assaultive violence.

The NHDS collects data from a sample of nonfederal, short-stay hospitals by discharge diagnosis and type of surgical procedures performed. The NHDS has been conducted annually since 1965 and is based on data abstracted from approximately 200,000 records from a sample of about 400 hospitals. Its findings are published in Series 13 of the Vital and Health Statistics Series. Data are available on hospital visits due to traumatic injury. However, these data are of limited value because (1) data on the cause of injury are not completely reported and vary greatly by the type of injury, and (2) the sample of hospitals is based only on those hospitals that agree to cooperate with the survey.

The NEISS is a surveillance system of injuries treated in hospital emergency rooms (ER) located throughout the United States. Currently, 66 hospitals contribute to NEISS. These hospitals represent a stratified probability sample of all hospitals with emergency rooms throughout the country and its territories, including hospitals with burn care centers using a 1985 sampling frame that stratified hospitals by size (number of ER visits). This system collects information on all injuries seen in the emergency room that could be deemed "product related," but not all products are included. For instance, automobile- and firearm-related injuries are not included in the list of products covered in the data collection system. NEISS could be expanded to collect information on morbidity and disability from assaultive violence.

State and Local Data Sources

Criminal Justice Agencies
State and local criminal justice agencies are a valuable source of data on assaultive violence. No federal laws require reporting to the FBI-UCR program, but 39 states have their own mandatory state reporting requirements. In such states, data from the state data collection agencies are forwarded to the FBI-UCR program. The agencies in the other 11 states report voluntarily to the UCR program. For example, since 1972 the State of Illinois has had mandatory UCR reporting on a statewide basis (21), has published their UCR data in an annual report entitled *Crime in Illinois* and has maintained a computerized database available for public use. County and city law enforcement agencies keep detailed records on crimes that come to their attention. These records, which ultimately form the bases for state- and national-level UCR data, are a potentially rich source of information on assaultive violence.

Coroner or Medical Examiner Records
Although coroner and medical examiner records are potentially useful sources of data for homicide, very few of these offices collect standardized

information on homicide deaths, and data from these offices are not collected or analyzed nationally. There is also considerable variation in the quality of information collected in various states. Whereas almost all states have medical examiners, few have medical examiners in each county, and records are often completed by persons acting as coroners. Data from coroner and medical examiner offices may be particularly useful for examining the relationship between alcohol and drug use and homicide victimization.

Medical and Social Service Agencies

Medical and social service agencies are another potentially valuable source of data on assaultive violence. Again, defintions and records concerning interpersonal violence have not been standardized, nor has there been any attempt to collect and analyze such data nationally. Even so, the records of agencies such as hospitals, battered women's shelters, mental health clinics, and substance abuse treatment facilities may contain a tremendous amount of useful information concerning the circumstances and histories of persons who have been victims or perpetrators of assaultive violence. A variety of methods have been developed to protect client confidentiality while allowing access to valuable data.

Needs for Improvement in Data Sources

Data on homicide both nationally and locally are generally considered to be fairly accurate. At the national level, FBI-UCR homicide data hold several advantages over the homicide data collected by NCHS from death certificates. First, FBI-UCR data are more timely than NCHS data because the FBI report is typically released nine to 10 months after the end of the calendar year being reported, whereas NCHS data are released two and one-half to three years after the reported year. Second, the FBI-UCR homicide data contain information on several critical variables that are not present in NCHS homicide data, such as the victim-offender relationship and circumstance and motives for the homicide. However, NCHS homicide data are generally considered to be more accurate and complete than FBI-UCR data. A comparison of FBI-UCR and NCHS homicide data for the period 1933–1975 revealed that the percentage of difference in the number of homicides identified in the two data sets averaged 7 percent a year, but was smaller in more recent years (10).

FBI-UCR data on homicide could be improved by establishing mandatory reporting requirements for all law enforcement agencies and instituting measures to insure that law enforcement agencies provide homicide information that is as complete as possible. NCHS vital data on homicide could be improved by amending the ICD E-codes and/or death certificates to include information such as the victim-offender relationship and to allow for the distinction between criminal and justifiable homicides. Such changes would increase the comparability and utility of these homicide data sources.

Data needs are much greater for nonfatal assaultive violence than for homicide. First, there is an urgent need at both the national and local levels for better information on injuries resulting from nonfatal assaults. Second, there is a need to develop systems that collect accurate information on the magnitude and nature of nonfatal assaultive violence between persons known to one another (e.g., family members, intimates, friends, and acquaintances). This is a particularly difficult task, and at present sources of such information have only limited utility for epidemiologic research and surveillance at the national and local levels.

These gaps in the availability of accurate information on assaultive violence must be filled if efforts at prevention in these areas are to advance. This need is particularly great at state and local levels. Such systems should establish as accurately as possible the extent and nature of interpersonal violence so that researchers and policymakers can (1) assess the impact of the problem, (2) determine the quality and type of resources needed to respond to the problem, and (3) develop baseline data that can help track the effectiveness of existing as well as new prevention and intervention strategies.

CAUSES AND RISK FACTORS

Current understanding of the causes and risk factors for assaultive violence is very rudimentary, but this section examines some of the more prominent theories of causation and research on risk factors found to be associated with fatal assaultive violence or homicide.

Theories on Causation

There are many types of assaultive violence and for each type the causes are complex and diverse. For this review, traditionally separate disciplinary approaches to understanding various aspects of the problem are summarized because each contributes valuable perspectives. Unfortunately, however, these separate approaches obscure the complex interaction of different types of factors that contribute to assaultive violence. Ultimately what is needed and what will prove most useful are causal explanations that combine biological, psychological, and sociological factors in ways that more clearly explain the occurrence of assaultive violence involving different perpetrators, victims, and circumstances.

Biological explanations of assaultive violence have examined gender, age, and certain psychiatric illnesses as important risk factors for homicide victimization and perpetration (22). With regard to gender, for example, it has been hypothesized that the marked preponderence of men among perpetrators and victims reflects the influence of male sex hormones on aggressive behavior. For example, the level of testosterone in the blood may immediately influence aggressive behavior, or the level of circulating sex hormones may influence the development of the fetal brain in ways that determine later propensities toward violence (22). In the case of the diminishing risk of victimization and perpetration associated with age, researchers have hypothesized that manifestations of overt aggression diminish with age as a result of biological transformations associated with aging (23).

Social learning theory and developmental theory are two major *psychological approaches* to violence. Social learning theory posits that behavior is learned through imitation of role models and reinforced by rewards and punishments received in interaction with others (24). Developmental theory focuses on deterrents to violence in the form of early parent-child ties of love; childhood experiences relatively free of punitive discipline or abuse; and experiences that reinforce the child's attachments, minimize frustrations, and encourage flexible inner controls (25).

There are four major *sociological approaches* to understanding homicide: cultural (or subcultural), structural, interactionist, and economic. Again, these are not mutually exclusive explanations, but each contributes in an important way to our overall understanding of the problem. The cultural approach posits that violent behavior is the result of learned, shared values and behaviors that are specific to a given group and applied in recognizable situations. The basic causes are the norms and values, transmitted across generations, that are learned by members of this group. Certain subgroups exhibit higher rates of assaultive violence because they are participants in a subculture that has violence as a norm. The cultural approach has been challenged by critics who point to the frequency of violence in groups in which it is clearly not normative (e.g., the middle class) and to the fact that it tends to "blame the victim." The cultural approach points toward interventions designed to change the norms, values, typical behaviors, or beliefs of specific high-risk groups. Such changes might be accomplished, for example, through education or by changing media images of persons with whom target group members are likely to identify.

The structural approach holds that rates of assaultive violence are largely influenced by broad-scale social forces, such as poverty or lack of opportunity, that operate independently of human cognition. In one widely recognized formulation, violence and other "illegitimate" behaviors arise when persons are deprived of "legitimate" means and resources to realize culturally valued goals. This theory does not adequately explain, however, why conflicts arising from structural deprivation lead to violence in one situation and other behaviors, passivity for instance, in other situations (26).

The interactionist approach focuses on the nature of the interaction sequence as it escalates into violent behavior and describes the process through which assaultive violence occurs. This kind of inquiry has been used most frequently to describe family violence (27). One investigator of 70 assault-homicide events in California, for example, described a series of offender and victim "moves" as they related to each other's moves and to the reaction of the audience. From this, he derived a set of time-ordered stages that most of the transactions followed (28). Other research has shown that violence grows out of a series of provocative arguments that escalate to murder. The arguments often are threats to one's identity (especially sexual identity) and one's self-esteem. Interventions based on the interactionist approach may range from helping couples recognize and resolve conflicts to limiting immediate access to lethal agents.

The economic approach, otherwise referred to as deterrence theory or the theory of economic choice, represents a particularly important perspective on the causes of assaultive violence because it provides the basis for many current policies aimed at reducing homicides and assault. This perspective represents an extension by orthodox economists of the principles of micro-economic theory to illegal activity. The main thrust of this theory is that decisions to engage in criminal behavior (e.g., the perpetration of physical assaults) are based on rational considerations (29). That is to say, a person commits an offense because the outcome appears more valuable than the outcome of other activities in which he or she could invest time and re-sources (30). Thus some people commit assaults not because their motiva-tion differs from that of other people, but because their perceived benefits and costs differ. Advocates of this theory suggest, therefore, that in order to prevent assaults we must increase the perpetrator's perceived costs by in-creasing the certainty and severity of punishment for such crimes. However, in order that the "desired" choices are made, people must be fully aware of the benefits and costs associated with all the alternative courses of action available to them. This theory assumes that all people have an equal capacity to make rational judgments under all conditions and circum-stances. But in the case of people under the influence of alcohol or drugs, for example, the ability to make rational judgments may be impaired.

Each of these theories has been used to explain different dimensions of assaultive violence. For example, in explaining the particularly high homicide rates for young black men, the following explanations have been offered (31):

1. *The subculture of violence.* Young blacks live in a cultural milieu that encourages violent solutions to problems, and culture is the mode of trans-mitting these norms from generation to generation. This subculture may have evolved from social and historical conditions in effect for many genera-tions (such as poverty and discrimination), but the cultural norms have now become somewhat independent of those conditions.

2. *The structure of society* (a structuralist interpretation). Young black men occupy a position in society in which they are deprived of opportunities for economic advancement, career satisfaction, and personal development. This deprivation leads to frustration and a search for alternative means of growth, individuation, and achievement. These alternative means frequently involve violent ends.

Factors Associated with Homicide

In the absence of a simple theory of causation for homicide, it is useful to review the factors that have been found or suggested to be associated with homicide based on empirical research. Knowledge of these factors is useful for targeting research and constructing preventive interventions.

Poverty is a structural factor associated with murders of friends and acquaintances, children, and spouses, and with robbery-associated murders of strangers (32–35). According to one study, it is more strongly associated with murders of family members and friends than murders of acquaintances (34). Two more structural factors, belief in male dominance and racial discrimination, are linked with killings of strangers and friends or acquaintances (32,36,37). Spouse homicides are associated with belief in male dominance (23,32,37).

Alcohol and drug consumption (an interactionist factor) have been associated with (but not shown to be a cause of) all types of homicide except child homicides. Many studies that have used histories of alcohol use by victim and/or perpetrator or victims' postmortem blood-alcohol concentrations have shown that about half of all victims and perpetrators had consumed alcohol before the homicide. However, without control or comparison populations, these studies have not been able to demonstrate a causal role for alcohol (38). The same situation applies to the association between alcohol use and family violence. For example, many violent adults abuse their spouses regardless of alcohol consumption. In addition, some researchers have suggested that, for many abusers, the disinhibiting effect of alcohol may be more psychological than physiological and that alcohol may serve as an excuse for behavior already decided upon (39).

In theory, alcohol and drug use may contribute to homicide by influencing the risk of both victimization and perpetration in a variety of ways. For example, alcohol use could be associated with victimization if it has a physiological effect on the brain that reduces inhibitions against aggressive behavior, thereby increasing the likelihood of an individual precipitating a life-threatening dispute. If so, alcohol and drug use may play an important role in what has been termed victim-precipitated homicide (38). Alternatively, alcohol and drug use may be associated with homicide victimization, not because of their physiological effects, but because their use is associated with specific situations, environments, or activities that place individuals at high risk for victimization. For example, drinking alcohol in a bar would place one at greater risk of victimization if bars attracted people who are more likely than the average person to behave violently toward others. Moreover, individuals who take illicit drugs, distribute them, or do both may have higher risks for homicide victimization because of the high profits, criminal behaviors, and instability associated with drug dealing (40). Thus these high risks of victimization might not be a direct consequence of the drug's biologic properties.

Other factors that predispose a person to homicide are listed in Figures 2-1 through 2-4. These diagrams are provided as a heuristic device for developing preventive interventions. The listings of factors are not meant to be all-inclusive. Only those factors are listed for which supportive empirical data have been cited in the literature on homicide, and, for some factors, the

Factors (Broad-scale social)

Structural	Cultural	Interactionist	Biological
• Poverty (32–35)	• Male belief in physical prowess, toughness, search for thrills and action (32,35)	• Drug and alcohol consumption (23,39,43,44)	• Male sex (23,32)
• Ideology that masculinity means a dominant male social role (23,32,36–37)	• Underdeveloped verbal skills (32)	• Weapons possession (43–48)	• Youth (20–29 years of age) (46,48,49)
• Racial segregation and discrimination (23,32,33,35,36,41)	• Belief that one should not intervene in another's fights (23)		
	• Televised violence and media support (42)		
	• Encouragement of fighting by bystanders (23)		

Prevention Strategies

Structural	Cultural	Interactionist
• Eliminate poverty and unemployment	• Reduce media violence	• Reduce alcohol and drug consumption
• Change conceptions of masculinity	• Increase community and witness intolerance for violence	• Reduce firearm injuries
• Reduce racial segregation and discrimination		• Teach conflict resolution skills for young men

Figure 2-1. Factors That May Predispose a Person to Kill a Friend or Acquaintance, and Possible Prevention Strategies.

Factors (Broad-scale social)

Structural	Cultural	Interactionist	Biological	Psychosocial
• Poverty and/or unemployment	• Belief in violence and/or physical punishment as socializing agent (50,51)	• Lack of adequate support facilities	• Young parental age	• Parents abused as children
• Too many and/or unintended pregnancies or children	• Belief that parents have ultimate right to do what they want with child		• Physical or mental disabilities of child	• Parents had violent role models
• Lack of education about child rearing	• Parents' unrealistic expectations of children (especially for children with mental or physical disabilities)			
• Parental dominance ideology (see cultural beliefs)				
• Prolonged marital stress				
• Social isolation nuclear family				

Prevention Strategies

Structural	Cultural	Interactionist	Biological	Psychosocial
• Eliminate poverty from families	• Establish alternate ways to socialize child	• Establish community/neighborhood intervention centers and hot-lines	• Prevent/treat childhood disabilities	• Treat identified abused children
• Reduce isolation of nuclear family	• Provide high-quality child-care facilities to reduce parental stress			
• Educate about planned parenthood and child rearing	• Aid handicapped children			
	• Change parental expectations of children			

Figure 2-2. Factors That May Predispose a Person to Kill or Abuse a Child, and Possible Prevention Strategies.

Model partially adopted from Richard Gelles (50), "Child Abuse as Psychopathology: A Sociological Critique and Reformulation." *Am J Orthopsychiatry* 1973; 43:611–621. Which factors distinguish between child abuse and killing of a child is unknown.

Factors (Broad-scale social)

Structural	Cultural	Interactionist
• Poverty (32–35)	• Male belief in physical prowess, toughness, that he is "head of house" and has control	• Alcohol and drug consumption (39,23,43,44)
• Masculine dominance over females (23,32,36,37)	• "Hands-off" view of domestic disputes by criminal justice system (52,53)	• Weapons possession (45–48)
• Isolation of nuclear family (39)	• Televised violence and other media supports (42)	• Male use of force to compensate for verbal disadvantage (32)
		• No safe place for women to go

Prevention Strategies

Structural	Cultural	Interactionist
• Eliminate poverty for men and women	• Increase verbal ability and means of problem-solving	• Reduce alcohol and drug consumption
• Eliminate sexual inequality (especially in child rearing and employment) and notions that masculinity requires dominance	• Initiate criminal-justice and social-service interventions	• Reduce firearm injuries
• Reduce isolation of nuclear family	• Reduce media violence	• Teach how to "fight fair" and resolve conflicts nonviolently
		• Teach how to walk away from a potentially violent situation
		• Increase availability of shelters

Figure 2-3. Factors That May Predispose a Person to Kill His/Her Spouse, and Possible Prevention Strategies.

Factors (Broad-scale social)

Structural	Cultural	Interactionist	Biological	Psychosocial
• Poverty (32–35)	• Materialism	• Lack of criminal-justice and legal prosecution (57)	• Male sex (23,32)	• Disorganized home life
• Ideology that masculinity means a dominant male social role (23,32,36,37)	• Male belief in thrills and action (32,55,56)	• Alcohol and drug consumption (23,39,43,44)	• Youth (teenagers) (46,48,49)	• Developmental lack in empathy (25)
• Racial segregation and discimination (23,32,33,35,36,41)	• Belief that perpetrator will not be caught or severely punished (57)	• Weapons possession (45–48)		
• Lack of role for adolescents	• Criminal way of life condoned, and opportunities provided to engage in it (58)			
• Urban density (population) (34,48,54)	• Belief that victims are not real and are to be used			
	• Externalization of blame			
	• Televised violence and media support for "bad guy" (42)			

Figure 2-4. Factors that may Predispose a Person to Commit a Robbery-Motivated Killing.

Prevention Strategies

Structural	Cultural	Interactionist
• Reduce poverty	• Reduce media violence	• Reduce alcohol and drug consumption
• Reduce racial segregation and urban density	• Increase empathy	• Reduce firearm injuries
• Create integrated, meaningful role for adolescents	• Increase community intolerance for robbery	• Educate potential victims
	• Increase swift, sure criminal-justice response to robbery and special handling of offenders who injure	• Initiate witness cooperation and assistance programs
		• Have "defensible space construction" (i.e., light up streets; construct safer places)
		• Initiate new patterns of police surveillance

Figure 2-5. Possible Prevention Strategies for a Person Who May Commit a Robbery-Motivated Killing.

evidence is stronger than for others. All factors are not equally important, but we have not attempted to assign them weights. Finally, the selection of category headings for these lists of factors was somewhat arbitrary, but categories were chosen to reflect the type of approach that gives greatest attention to a particular factor. Obviously, some factors figure importantly in several different approaches and could be listed under any of several headings.

OUTCOMES

Mortality

In 1986 homicides in the United States accounted for the loss of at least 21,731 lives based on NCHS mortality data. Overall, these deaths accounted for more than 650,000 potential years of life lost, an index in which homicide ranked fourth among all causes of death. Homicide was the twelfth leading cause of death for Americans; for young black people (15–34 years old), homicide was *the* leading cause of death. The United States, in fact, has one of the highest homicide rates of any country in the world when compared with other countries that report homicide statistics to the World Health Organization (Table 2-1) (59). In comparing homicide rates from different countries, it must be noted that reporting methods may differ and that domestic and international wars may affect homicide rates in some areas.

Demographic Patterns

Homicide takes its greatest toll among minorities, men, and the young. For the average American in 1980, the lifetime probability of murder victimization was one out of 153; for white American women, one out of 450; for a black man, one out of 28 (4). For a young black man, 20–24 years old, the odds are greater than one out of three that if he dies, his death will be due to homicide. It is difficult to disentangle the contribution of race from socioeconomic status in explaining the high homicide rates among black men, but several studies suggest that socioeconomic status is the more important determinant (60,61).

Ethnicity also appears to be an important determinant of homicide rates. An analysis of mortality data collected for the period 1976–1980 by the health departments of five southwestern states—in which more than 60 percent of all Hispanics in the United States reside—showed the overall homicide rate for Hispanics (20.5 per 100,000) was more than two and one-half times the Anglo (non-Hispanic whites) rate (7.9 per 100,000). The overall homicide rate for Hispanic men (36.7 per 100,000) was more than three times the rate for Anglo men (11.7 per 100,000). This difference was most striking in the younger male age groups in which the Hispanic homicide rate was almost five times that for Anglos (62).

Table 2-1 Deaths from Homicide and Injury Purposefully Inflicted by Other Persons (Rate per 100,000 Population, 1985)

Country	All Ages Men	All Ages Women	Men 15–24	Men 25–34	Absolute Number
Puerto Rico	30.6	3.6	44.8	64.9	579
Paraguay	13.6	1.8	16.0	28.0	182
United States	12.7	3.9	18.5	22.6	19,628
Panama	9.4	1.0	15.4	15.5	115
Guatemala (1984)	5.3	1.3	4.1	15.1	256
Costa Rica	7.9	1.8	10.5	13.7	127
Barbados (1984)	7.5	3.0	—	14.0	13
Suriname	7.5	3.2	9.3	12.4	20
Northern Ireland	6.6	1.0	10.3	11.3	58
Chile	5.7	0.8	6.4	10.8	387
Bulgaria	4.6	1.8	5.1	6.4	289
Singapore	3.5	1.4	4.5	6.8	62
Hungary	3.2	2.1	2.4	3.6	283
Israel	2.9	1.4	3.5	6.2	91
Kuwait	2.8	0.7	6.6	2.2	32
Canada	2.7	1.5	3.1	4.9	537
Australia	2.5	1.5	3.4	3.3	314
New Zealand	2.5	1.6	5.6	2.7	66
Iceland	2.5	—	4.6	4.9	3
Italy	2.4	0.6	2.9	4.5	841
Yugoslavia	2.3	1.2	2.2	3.1	401
Luxembourg	2.2	1.1	—	6.7	6
Scotland	1.9	0.8	3.3	3.5	69
Denmark*	1.8	1.1	1.7	2.6	74
Hong Kong	1.7	1.2	1.5	2.6	80
Sweden*	1.7	0.8	1.3	2.2	104
France	1.7	0.9	1.2	2.5	694
Austria	1.6	1.2	0.9	2.2	107
Greece	1.5	0.6	1.4	2.5	106
Switzerland*	1.2	1.6	1.4	1.0	93
Germany, Federal Republic of	1.2	1.1	0.9	1.4	726
Norway*	1.2	0.7	1.5	2.8	40
Netherlands	1.2	0.5	0.6	2.7	126
Japan	1.0	0.7	0.3	0.7	1,017
England and Wales	0.8	0.6	0.8	0.9	344
Ireland	0.7	0.6	0.6	2.0	23
Mauritius	0.6	0.6	—	2.3	6

*Deaths classified by 8th version of International Classification of Diseases (ICD); all other countries used 9th version of ICD.

Source: World Health Organization Statistics Annuals, 1986, 1987, and 1988 (59)

Victim-Offender Relationship

Of the homicides committed in the United States in 1986 and reported to the FBI, 40.0 percent involved friends and acquaintances; 15.1 percent were within families; and 12.5 percent were between strangers (63) (Table 2-2). The category of "relationship unknown" accounted for 32.4 percent of

Table 2-2 Number of Homicide Deaths and Rates per 100,000 Population by Race, Sex, and Relationahip, 1986

| | White | | | | | | Black and Other | | | | | | Race/Sex | Total | | % of |
| | Men | | Women | | Total | | Men | | Women | | Total | | Unknown | | | Homicides |
Relationship	Rate	(No.)	Rate	(No.)	Rate	(No.)	Rate	(No.)	Rate	(No.)	Rate	(No.)		Rate	(No.)	
Family	0.8	(816)	0.8	(882)	0.8	(1,698)	4.3	(759)	2.5	(487)	3.4	(1,246)	5	1.2	(2,949)	15.1
Friend	3.0	(3,000)	0.8	(875)	1.9	(3,875)	18.2	(3,189)	3.8	(738)	10.7	(3,927)	20	3.2	(7,822)	40.0
Stranger	1.2	(1,241)	0.3	(263)	0.7	(1,504)	4.6	(812)	0.6	(115)	2.5	(927)	5	1.0	(2,436)	12.5
Unknown	2.4	(2,412)	0.9	(898)	1.6	(3,310)	13.5	(2,369)	3.0	(578)	8.0	(2,947)	69	2.6	(6,326)	32.4
Total	7.5	(7,419)	2.8	(2,981)	5.1	(10,387)	40.6	(7,129)	10.0	(1,918)	24.6	(9,047)	98	8.6	(20,613)[a]	100.0%

[a]A total of 20,613 murder and nonnegligent manslaughter victims and justifiable homicide victims were reported to the FBI-UCR program in 1986.

homicides. However, data suggest that many homicides classified as "relationship unknown" are most likely to be murders of strangers because murders that occur between intimates are more likely to be cleared (i.e., an arrest is made) and appropriately classified.

Most family homicides involve spouses and occur in the home. They frequently occur after many assaultive incidents (28,39). The median age of victims is 33 and of offenders, 32. In 38.4 percent of the cases, a handgun is used, followed by other guns (19.5%), knives (17.0%), and other means (25.1%).

Victims of acquaintance homicide are typically younger than the victims of family homicide and much more likely to be male and black. This type of homicide is more prevalent among blacks and races other than white (43.4% of the victims in 1986) than among whites (37.3% in 1986). Offenders (median age 23) are usually younger than their victims. Handguns, again the weapon of choice, are used in 44.7 percent of the cases; knives, in 19.5 percent. Homicides involving friends are most likely to occur within a private residence, although one-third occur on the street, and a higher percentage occurs in bars than is true for other types of killings (36).

In stranger homicides, the victims and offenders are predominantly male and the median age of the victim (31 years) is higher than that of the offender (25 years). Most such killings are with firearms (49.1% with handguns, 12.2% with another type of gun). Nationally, 46.9 percent of such killings are associated with another crime, often robbery. In cities, most stranger killings (57%) are associated with another crime, most frequently with robbery (36). Despite such figures and the fact that robbery murders increased in the 1970s (47,48), the chance of being killed in a robbery remains relatively small.

In those instances where the relationship of the murderer to the victim was known, murder by a friend or acquaintance accounted for the greatest number of homicide deaths (7,822), a rate of 3.2 per 100,000. Murder by a member of the victim's family accounted for 2,949 deaths (1.2 per 100,000) (Table 2.2). Of all the homicides committed in 1986, 55.1 percent were committed by individuals known to their victims and more than one-quarter of those were committed by family members.

Homicide Weapons
In 1986, 59.1 percent of homicides were committed with firearms. Of those homicide victims, almost three-quarters (74.1%) were killed with handguns. After firearms, cutting and piercing instruments were the next most frequently used weapon (20.3%), followed by bodily force (6.7%) and blunt objects (5.6%) (Fig. 2-6). Other or undetermined weapons accounted for 8.3 percent of homicides in 1986.

Circumstance
Homicide deaths may be classified according to whether victims were killed during the commission of another felony (e.g., robbery) or whether they occurred during nonfelony circumstances (e.g., an argument). A relatively

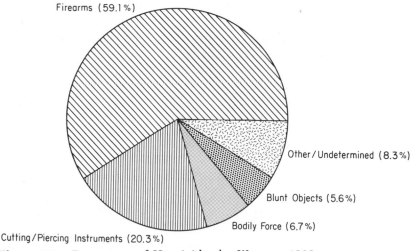

Firearms (59.1%)

Other/Undetermined (8.3%)

Blunt Objects (5.6%)

Bodily Force (6.7%)

Cutting/Piercing Instruments (20.3%)

Figure 2-6. Percentage of Homicides by Weapon, 1986.

small proportion of homicides are committed during the perpetration of another felony or crime. In 1986 only 19.4 percent of homicides that occurred in the United States were committed during the course of another crime such as robbery or narcotics offenses. The most frequently occurring circumstance associated with homicide is verbal argument. In 1986, 37.5 percent of homicides were associated with verbal arguments. Other nonfelony circumstances including brawls due to the influence of alcohol or narcotics, juvenile gang killings, and institutional killings, for example, accounted for 18.6 percent of the circumstances associated with homicide. In 22.5 percent of the cases, the circumstances leading to the killing were unknown.

Morbidity

Data from the National Crime Survey on violent crimes provide a partial measure of the morbidity associated with assaultive violence. For Americans over the age of twelve, 5.5 million incidents of violent crime (i.e., simple and aggravated assault, robbery, and rape) occurred in 1986 (19). This figure represents a rate of 2,810 violent crimes per 100,000 people age 12 and over (19). Simple and aggravated assaults accounted for 79.3 percent of these incidents of assaultive violence. Attempted and completed robbery accounted for 18.3 percent of these incidents; attempted and completed rape accounted for the remaining 2.4 percent. Men were 1.7 times more likely to be victims than females, with men ages 16–19 being at greatest risk (8,120 per 100,000) (19). Blacks were at 1.2 times greater risk of being a victim of a violent crime than whites; Hispanics were about equally likely as non-Hispanics to have been a victim (19).

Almost one-third of victims (32.2%) of robbery and assault sustained a physical injury. Given the severe emotional trauma associated with rape, all victims are considered to have been injured regardless of whether or not a physical injury was reported. Of all violent crime victims, 7.8 percent received hospital care. Hospital costs (for those who survived assaults plus those who eventually died as a result of aggravated assault) totaled approximately $606 million. The cost of physician visits raised that figure to $638 million. No data are available for the costs of emergency room treatment, pharmaceuticals, extended care after initial hospitalization, or the treatment of offenders who were injured in aggravated assaults.

Aggravated assaults accounted for more than 8 million days lost from activities such as paid work, school, or child rearing: at least 4,718,200 of those were paid workdays. Because a large percentage of victims are women who are economically dependent on their husbands, it is likely that a great deal of time was lost from major nonpaying activity such as child care and housekeeping. The "costs" of assaultive violence should also include time lost by children from school or preschool because of domestic violence, child abuse, and neglect, but data are not available to allow these estimates. Assaults may result in a wide range of possible disabilities, primarily psychological, sensory, and musculoskeletal. The average cost of losing one's vision or of the incapacitating fear that prevents one from returning home after a life-threatening attack that has taken place there is incalculable.

Projections based on the National Crime Society indicate that from 1982 to 1984 there were approximately 1,502,400 incidents of assaultive violence (i.e., rape, robbery, aggravated assault, simple assault) perpetrated by family members, a rate of 213.8 per 100,000 U.S. population (not the population within those families) (64). Other estimates of the number of women beaten each year range from 1.8 million (65) to 3–4 million (66). Assaults within families represent at least 21,000 hospitalizations, 99,800 hospital days, 28,700 emergency room visits, and 39,900 physician visits. Health care costs incurred for domestic assaults totaled at least $44,393,700.

Assaults within families accounted for at least 175,500 days lost from paid work in 1980. Although the injuries suffered by abused women do not typically result in hospitalization, many of them do. More important than the cost of hospitalization, however, is the enormous drain on medical resources. Battered women, who frequently use medical services in lieu of other refuge, present myriad complaints lacking evidence of specific disease and, during a lifetime, may make hundreds of visits because of abuse. Of all the emergency room visits made by women seeking treatment for injury, 19 percent involved battering. Battered women use medical and psychiatric services many times more frequently than other women, and visits motivated by battering may be even more common at such primary care sites as the maternity clinic or ambulatory care service (66).

Quality of Life

Assaultive violence affects victims, their families, and society as a whole. An assault may result in only a minor physical injury but may have a devastating impact upon the victim's life in terms of fear, anxiety, and subsequent restrictions in activities and movements. Victims of actual attacks and victims of fear may become quite isolated, and the changes they make in job, home, or patterns of activities may markedly constrict their freedom and lower the quality of their lives. The changes they make in their jobs or homes to increase the sense of personal security constantly remind them of the new fears and restrictions that have become part of their lives. Homicide can have a crippling effect on surviving family members that affects several generations.

Research indicates that children who are victims of violence suffer delays in physical, social, and emotional development. Many children who witness violence suffer from posttraumatic stress disorders, conditions frequently made worse when they must participate as an official witness in court (67). Similarly, battered women are at greatly elevated risk of alcoholism, drug abuse, attempted suicide, fear of child abuse, rape, and mental health problems, including severe depression and even psychosis (66). Family violence is one of the four most common reasons cited for divorce, and although divorce may solve the immediate problems, it may also result in increased economic deprivation for women and children. There is also considerable evidence that being divorced or single, in itself, does not protect women from subsequent battering. At one large metropolitan hospital, 72 percent of the women who had battering injuries were single, separated, or divorced (66).

The threat of violent attack may be as damaging as the attack itself. Battered spouses and children may focus all their energies on reducing the chance that a partner or parent will explode in violent rage, and it is impossible to calculate the potential achievements and creativity lost in such situations. The physical abuse of women may lead to child abuse, although the relationship of the two problems remains unclear. The health care system may contribute to volatile family situations by giving battered women unnecessary medications, inferior care, and labels that stigmatize.

Interpersonal violence lowers the quality of life in society as a whole by contributing to days lost from work and by exacting financial expenditures for police and criminal justice intervention, social service intervention, and emergency room and trauma center services. In addition, school systems must cope with children who are likely to have academic and social problems as a result of maltreatment at home. In families where battering occurs, the children, even if not physically abused, commonly suffer inordinate fear and anxiety, have frequent nightmares and enuresis, and "act out" (boys) or become passive (girls).

INTERVENTIONS TO PREVENT ASSAULTIVE VIOLENCE

A strategy to substantially reduce and prevent the incidence of assaultive violence must involve both broad social changes in our overall approach to violence and specific interventions aimed at cases of potential or actual violence, assault, or abuse. These specific interventions may try to reach individuals before a pattern of victimization or interpersonal violence is established, or they may attempt to minimize the consequences and costs of interpersonal violence by providing its victims with appropriate support and by helping perpetrators to change. However, our knowledge of how to prevent violence is far less extensive than our knowledge of its scope and impact. Few authors deal specifically with preventing assault or homicide. Only 17 of the 364 items in a 1982 bibliography on homicide deal with prevention (36).

As the Minneapolis police department demonstrated in its recent assessment of different approaches to spouse abuse, we need not wait to understand the complex causes of violence to engage in bold experiments to prevent it (68). Both the National Commission on Violence (25) and the attorney general's Task Force on Family Violence (69) have catalogued dozens of specific policy recommendations requiring local, state, and federal action. In addition, *Injury Prevention: Meeting the Challenge* (70) presents an extensive review of interventions to prevent interpersonal violence and summarizes what is known about the effectiveness of each one. These reports should be reviewed by all who wish to implement specific preventive interventions. The recommendations in this chapter are less detailed than these other reports; instead, they are grouped by sector and presented to suggest approaches that could be considered for implementation as a general public policy, health and social services, criminal justice, and environmental changes. Because the effectiveness of these interventions remains to be evaluated in most cases, these proposals are presented as options to be tried and tested.

Social and Cultural Changes

The aim of the following proposals is to change the social, cultural, and physical contexts most likely to evoke violent behavior.

1. *Decrease the cultural acceptance of violence.* Few people believe that violence is an appropriate way to settle disputes, but there is widespread tolerance for violence among and/or against certain groups (blacks, teenagers, women, children). These forms of violence may frequently be rationalized or tolerated as impulsive behaviors evoked by competition, jealousy, or threats to personal authority and identity. Public health education must target these widespread beliefs and promote the notion that violent individuals are responsible for their behavior. Community resources should be mobilized to make it clear that interpersonal violence is a problem that can be addressed and not an inalterable fact of life. Specific attention should be given to evaluating the portrayal of violence in children's television programming and the role of corporal punishment at schools and in homes.

2. *Reduce racial discrimination and the effects of racism.* In young black men, the cultural acceptance of violence has been linked with low self-esteem and low valuations of human life, especially that of other blacks. These low valuations of oneself and others have been associated with racism and limited access to social and economic resources.

3. *Reduce gender inequality and support more flexible male role models.* Conflicts over limited resources and unequal responsibility based on gender are an important source of violence among family and intimates. Male role models should emphasize flexibility, shared decision making, and non-violent means of self-development and expression.

4. *Reduce the consumption of alcohol and other drugs.* The use or abuse of alcohol and other drugs has been associated with all forms of violence, even though clear cause and effect relationships have not yet been shown. Interventions sensitive to the peer pressures and cultural contexts in which substance abuse develops should be geared particularly toward adolescents and young adults and should emphasize the benefits of dependence-free development as well as the effects of harmful substances on self-control. Prevention can also focus on environmental changes such as raising the minimum drinking age, passing stricter laws against driving while intoxicated, limiting the hours and places where alcohol can be served, and regulating alcohol advertising.

Health and Related Social Services

1. *Develop educational programs to teach conflict-resolution skills.* Schools, churches, health-care providers, and other community agencies and institutions could offer educational programs to teach conflict resolution skills. Special programs might be developed for high-risk populations, such as black, male adolescents, focusing on the magnitude of the threat that homicide and assault pose to lives and health, how to recognize volatile situations before they escalate, and how to diffuse or walk away from potentially homicidal fights (71,72). Health educators should review what is current in this area, evaluate those programs already in existence, design new approaches, and field-test and evaluate these new curricula.

2. *Increase education for family life, family planning, and child rearing.* Education in these three areas appears to hold considerable promise for reducing family stress and violence (73). Family planning information and services would reduce the incidence of unwanted or unexpected children born into families that have neither the inclination nor the resources to cope with these children.

Parent and family-life education programs that serve all parents avoid the problem of having to identify at-risk families; therefore, such curricula, which would include preventive education as well as education about reporting physical and sexual abuse, should be integrated into grades K–12 of the public school system (74). Reducing violence in the home might reduce the amount of violence learned there and later perpetrated against acquaintances and strangers. Family education about developmental difficulties might help parents identify and seek appropriate treatments for children with aggressive and antisocial behaviors.

3. *Support families with community-based support services.* Research indicates that individuals and families embedded in kin and community groups are less likely to be abusive than individuals who are socially and/or physically isolated (39,65,75). Therefore, federal, state, and local governments should try to enhance the development of grassroots groups and organizations that serve to integrate individuals into the community. These groups should target their programs to adults, youth, and families. Tax, welfare, and business policies that promote isolation and divide families should also be reexamined.

4. *Address and remedy problems in the recognition of cases of violence.* The medical care system frequently fails to recognize the etiology of injuries that are the result of assaults, fails to report such incidents even when reporting is mandated, and thus fails to identify individuals at high risk for subsequent injuries. Risk profiles and a history of victimization or perpetration of violence should be made part of every physical examination.

5. *Decrease disincentives for medical personnel to become involved.* The legal entanglements that surround cases of child and woman abuse, as well as the exposure to threats of violence against themselves, often prevent health care personnel from even questioning their patients about the cause of their injuries. If such instances of violence are to be stopped, these disincentives need to be addressed. One example of an intervention that might penetrate these barriers is special child- and assault-trauma intervention teams that combine the disciplines of social work, psychiatry, gynecology, and pediatrics.

6. *Improve the management and treatment of victims of violence.* The medical care system often fails to adequately intervene in or follow up on cases of traumatic injury from violent assaults. This is particularly necessary with high-risk groups, such as infants or adolescents, who may be in danger of repeated attacks or homicide. Trauma or crisis treatment centers should offer victims of assaultive violence the same range of services that are provided to rape victims, for example, because these victims are frequently traumatized psychologically as well as physically. Community-based trauma treatment centers should also offer comprehensive care designed to involve high-risk individuals in ongoing prevention-oriented programs.

7. *Improve the ability of the health care system to recognize and treat consequences of violence other than injuries.* These consequences include alcoholism, drug dependency, and psychiatric trauma. Particularly urgent is the need for intervention programs for children who are victims of violence (including physical assault, incest, and sexual abuse), as well as for those who witness violence (such as a murder, rape, or suicide of a parent) (67). Witnesses of violence need help dealing with the criminal justice system because their experience as witnesses may traumatize them further. Shelters

for battered women may be an important model for providing comprehensive services to victims of other types of violence.

8. *Decrease financial barriers to care for victims.* Ensure that victims can receive medical care without being dependent upon adequate medical insurance.

9. *Improve the identification and treatment of perpetrators of violence by the health care system.* Since perpetrators of violence are themselves often injured, they frequently require health services, making this an important entry point for identification and treatment.

10. *Improve record-keeping and reporting for victims of interpersonal violence.* Health care institutions and personnel, for example, frequently do not comply with state laws requiring reporting of gunshot wounds. This type of information may be critical to assess the effectiveness of the health-care system's response to violence.

11. *Improve communication and cooperation among health care providers, police departments, and schools.* The health care sector—including hospitals—needs to keep records of violent incidents and report them to the appropriate agencies. This is important not only in identifying individuals at risk, but also as documentation for victims who later may decide to prosecute. Linking data available in the health care sector with police data may also be helpful in identifying high-risk individuals and setting up intervention programs (76). Health professionals should also work with educators to develop health education curricula that address issues of self-directed and interpersonal violence.

12. *Develop programs to train high-risk adolescents and to make jobs available for them.* "Adolescent marginality" is a term that sociologists use to identify a risk factor for violence. It refers to the lack of integration and of a clear, positive role for adolescents in our culture. If violence is to be reduced among the young where its incidence is too high, we need to focus our attention on this factor.

13. *Focus on prevention in the treatment of illness related to consumption of alcohol and other drugs.* Health care personnel interact with many abusers of these substances, concentrating on immediate problems like overdoses or detoxification, and sometimes on less important problems like bruises. In their concern for immediate problems, however, they often fail to address issues of prevention.

Criminal Justice Changes

Changes in the criminal justice system focus on the police and the courts. The first four of the possible interventions that follow concern the police or more active citizen interaction with the police. The other major arm of the criminal justice system involves the courts and lawmakers, prosecutors, and prisons. Attempts in these systems to deal with homicide have usually taken two forms: *deterrence* (establishing and imposing more sanctions, thereby hoping to deter others) and *incapacitation* (physically restraining offenders, thereby preventing them from committing other crimes). Despite the vast number of studies on deterrence and incapacitation, however, the effect of different sanctions on various crime types is largely unknown (77).

1. *Police should treat physical assaults among family members, intimates, and acquaintances as criminal behavior.* Police should not fail to pursue and prosecute assaultive violence merely because the victim and perpetrator know each other. Milder forms of family and acquaintance violence may escalate to forms as lethal and severe as any type of assaultive violence between strangers (65,78).

2. *Train police and citizen intervention teams.* When called to a dispute, police have typically responded either by trying to address only the immediate situation or by making an arrest. The number of repeat calls would indicate that they have been ineffective in quelling such disturbances. In 1967 the New York City Police Department tried another approach: the Family Crisis Intervention Unit. In this experiment, specially trained officers were taught to mediate disputes and refer troubled people to other social service agencies. Although the results did not document a precise reduction in family homicides, they did illustrate that changes in police intervention can reduce family assaults as well as injuries to police officers and to increase referrals to social service agencies (20% of the 75% referred actually sought help) (37).

Generally, few police departments have such programs, so extending this practice should take high priority. Such teams need to be very sensitive to the concerns of women and minorities if they are going to reduce rather than potentially increase the violence. Crisis intervention units run by nonpolice may be even more effective than police-staffed units. There are three types of nonpolice units: those located within the police complex although administered by civilian personnel; units located with City Hall (or, as in Dade County, Florida, for example, a prosecutor's office) that work in close conjunction with the police and other emergency services; and units that are community-based with some form of direct access to police and other emergency services. Local conditions determine the best application of the concept. In addition to providing backup to the police where rape and assault victims or the relatives of homicide victims require support, such crisis units may serve a preventive function if called to situations before disputes break into violence or when participants in quarrels would prefer nonpolice resolution. Police departments frequently collect tremendous amounts of information on domestic calls, so this information could be used by crisis intervention teams to identify high-risk individuals and families. These individuals could then be given priority in the delivery of specific services. Such records could also be used to identify general risk factors for serious domestic violence and to evaluate the effectiveness of intervention teams and the police. Finally, the extrapolation of this method of intervention to other dispute situations, such as those between friends and neighbors, might be profitable.

3. *Improve linkages between police and social services in response to violence.* For many poor and persons at high risk of victimization or perpetration of violence, particularly women and blacks, the police are the only service agency with which they come in contact. It is important that the police be able to appropriately and effectively refer these people to health and social service agencies that are willing and capable of providing needed services.

4. *Initiate informal citizen surveillance and silent-witness programs.* Police patrol capabilities can be extended by informal citizen surveillance. The Violence Center at the University of Pennsylvania evaluated all such programs and found that most town watches focus on burglary, disorderly conduct, and robbery, not on homicide. Uncontrolled studies report decreases (often substantial) in burglary once the town watch is in place. Similar citizen surveillance strategies for interpersonal violence might help reduce homicides because of the advantages of more rapid citizen response to disputes and increased reporting of child abuse.

Silent witness programs that provide help, support, and protection for those who testify can be extended to aid in apprehension and conviction. A Rand study of detectives found that most crimes, including homicides, are solved because someone witnessed the event, an informant told the police, or the victim identified the offender (79).

5. *Facilitate access of victims to legal services.* The courts should use protective orders, temporary restraining orders, and peace bonds to keep violent offenders from attacking partners or children. This access to legal services is especially needed in rural areas.

6. *Initiate victim and witness assistance programs.* Court processing for interpersonal violence cases needs to be accelerated so that there is not a long waiting period between the initial arrest and final disposition. Services should also be organized so that the victim does not have to return to court several times.

Environmental and Other Changes

In addition to changes in society and culture, in the delivery of health and related social services, and in the operation of our criminal justice system, certain adaptations of the environment have been proposed to deter violence.

1. *Develop strategies to reduce injuries associated with firearms.* In 1985, 31,566 persons died as a result of firearm injuries. Of these decedents, 17,363 died from suicide; 11,836 died from homicide; 1,649 died from unintentionally inflicted injuries; 242 died from homicide due to legal intervention; and for 476, the medicolegal cause of death was undetermined (80). Firearm mortality rates for females, male teenagers, and young adults have been higher during the 1980s than at any time previously (81).

Firearm injuries also appear to be an important cause of morbidity in the United States. National estimates of the extent and distribution of firearm morbidity, however, are grossly inadequate for determining the full extent of this problem. The most recent estimates from data collected in 1972 in the National Health Interview Survey indicate that for every fatality due to firearm injuries, there are at least five nonfatal injuries (82).

Despite the magnitude and costs of firearm injuries, scientific investigations in this area have only begun to scratch the surface of what we need to know about this problem. To the detriment of scientific inquiry, the role of firearms in producing injury and crime is an extremely contentious political and social issue in our society. If we are to discover effective strategies for preventing firearm injuries, however, we must avoid polemics and adopt a scientific perspective toward this issue.

Common approaches to the prevention of firearm injuries include: (1) strict licensing; (2) prohibitions against buying, selling, or possessing guns; (3) prohibitions against carrying (but not owning) guns; and (4) mandatory penalties for the use of a gun in a felony and for carrying unlicensed firearms. There is little scientific evidence to show definitely that legislative approaches such as those listed above are effective in controlling firearm injuries. Many countries where ownership of handguns is severely limited have homicide rates that are markedly below that of the United States (83), but these countries differ in other significant ways from the United States so that the difference in homicide rates cannot be attributed solely to laws governing the availability and access to handguns.

2. *Have "defensible space construction."* This ecological/sociological term refers to using architectural and social-planning principles to create safe environments. It covers everything from having well-lit courtyards in housing areas to having decent homes for all Americans.

3. *Define high-risk settings and occupations and determine interventions specific for them.* Police, prisoners, and cab drivers are three examples of groups at high risk of being assaulted or murdered. The use of bullet-proof vests or barriers for taxicab drivers, for example, could make their environs more safe and thus reduce their risk.

ACKNOWLEDGMENTS

We are grateful to many people for their significant contributions to the research and writing of this chapter. In particular, we would like to thank Evan Stark, Ph.D., Margaret A. Zahn, Ph.D., Richard J. Gelles, Ph.D., and Thomas Lalley, M.A., for their many suggestions and critiques. Special thanks to Donna Hiett for assistance in the preparation of this manuscript.

REFERENCES

1. Centers for Disease Control. Homicide surveillance: High-risk racial and ethnic groups—blacks and Hispanics, 1970 to 1983. Atlanta: Centers for Disease Control, 1986.

2. US Dept. of Justice, Bureau of Justice Statistics. Criminal victimization in the United States, 1986: A National Crime Survey report. Washington, DC: Bureau of Justice Statistics, US Dept. of Justice. (NCJ-111456), 1988.
3. O'Carroll PW, Mercy JA. Patterns and recent trends in black homicide. In: Hawkins DF, ed. Homicide among black Americans. Lanham, Maryland: University Press of America, 1986: 29–42.
4. US Dept. of Justice. Crime in the United States, 1981. Washington, DC: US Dept. of Justice, 1982.
5. National Center for Health Statistics. Advance report, final mortality statistics, 1980. Hyattsville, MD: National Center for Health Statistics, August 1983; DHHS pub. no. (PHS) 83-1120 (Monthly Vital Statistics Report; vol 23 no 5, supp.).
6. Kelsey JL, Thompson WD, Evans AS. Methods in observational epidemiology. New York: Oxford University Press, 1986.
7. Mercy JA, O'Carroll PW. New directions in violence prediction: The public health arena. Violence and Victims 1988; 3(4):285–301.
8. US Dept. of Justice. Crime in the United States, 1986. Washington, DC: US Dept. of Justice, 1987.
9. Barancik JI, Chatterjee BF, Greene YZ, Mekenzie EM, Fife B. Northeastern Ohio Trauma Study: I Magnitude of the problem. AJPH July 1983; 73(7):746–751.
10. Cantor D, Cohen LE. Comparing measures of homicide trends: Methodological and substantive differences in the Uniform Crime Report time series. Soc Sci Research 1980; 9:121–145.
11. Beattie RH. Criminal statistics in the United States—1960. J Crim Law, Criminol Police Sci 1960; 51:49–65.
12. Beattie RH. Problems of criminal statistics in the United States. In: Wolfgang ME, Savitz L, Johnston N, eds. The sociology of crime and delinquency. New York: Wiley, 1962.
13. Wolfgang ME. Uniform Crime Reports: A critical appraisal. University of Pennsylvania Law Review 1963; 72:708–738.
14. Robinson SM. A critical review of the Uniform Crime Reports. University of Michigan Law Review 1966; 64:1031–1054.
15. Lejins PP. Uniform Crime Reports. University of Michigan Law Review 1966; 6:1011–1030.
16. Savitz LD. Official police statistics and their limitations. In: Savitz LD, Hohnson N, eds. Crime in society. New York: Wiley, 1978.
17. Hindelang MJ. The Uniform Crime Reports revisited. J. Criminal Justice 1974; 2:1–17.
18. US Dept. of Justice, Bureau of Justice Statistics. National Crime Surveys: National Sample, 1973–1979, Ann Arbor. Michigan: Inter-University Consortium Political and Social Research, 1981.
19. Technical Notes. Hyattsville, MD: National Center for Health Statistics, 1989, (Monthly Vital Statistics Reports, appears in all issues).
20. US Dept. of Health and Human Services. International classification of diseases, 9th revision, clinical modification. Washington, DC: US Gov. Printing Office, 1980.
21. Illinois Criminal Justice Information Authority. Research bulletin-introduction to Illinois uniform crime reports. Illinois Criminal Justice Information Authority, May 1985.

22. Mednick SA, Pollock V, Volavka J, Gabrielli J. Biology and violence. In: Wolfgang ME, Weiner NA, eds. Criminal violence. Beverly Hills: Sage, 1982: 21–80.
23. Wolfgang ME. Patterns in criminal homicide. New York: Wiley, 1958.
24. Megargee EI. Psychological determinants and correlates of criminal violence. In: Weiner MA, ed. Criminal violence. Beverly Hills: Sage, 1982: 81–170.
25. Mulvihill DJ, Tunin MM, eds. Crimes of violence: A staff report submitted to the National Commission on the Causes and Prevention of Violence. Washington, DC: US Gov. Printing Office, 1969.
26. Wolfgang ME, Zahn MA. Criminal homicide. In: Kadish SH, ed. Encyclopedia of crime and justice. New York: Free Press, 1983.
27. Dobash RE, Dobash R. Violence against wives. New York: Free Press, 1979.
28. Luckenbill DF. Criminal homicide as a situated transaction. Soc Problems 1977; 25:176–186.
29. Rubin PH. The economics of crime. Atlanta Economic Review, July/August 1978; 28(4):38–43.
30. Becker G. Crime and punishment: An economic approach. J Political Economy, March 1968: 1169–1217.
31. Rose HM. The geography of despair. Annals Assoc Am Geographers 1978; 68:4.
32. Curtis LA. Violence, race and culture. Lexington, MA: D.C. Heath, 1975.
33. Rose HM. Lethal aspects of urban violence. Lexington, MA: D.C. Heath, 1979.
34. Smith MD, Parker RN. Type of homicide and variation in regional rates. Soc Forces 1980: 136–147.
35. Wolfgang ME, Ferracuti F. The subculture of violence: Towards an integrated theory in criminology. London: Tavistock, 1967.
36. Riedel M, Zahn MA. The nature and patterns of American homicide: An annotated bibliography. Washington, DC: National Institute of Justice, 1982.
37. Steinmetz SK, Straus MA. Violence in the family. New York: Harper and Row, 1974.
38. Goodman RA, Mercy JA, Loya F, Rosenberg ML, Smith JC, Allen NH, Vargas L, Kolts R. Alcohol use and interpersonal violence: Alcohol detected in homicide victims. American Journal of Public Health 1986; 76(2):144–149.
39. Gelles RJ. The violent home: A study of physical aggression between husbands and wives. Beverly Hills: Sage, 1974.
40. Goldstein PJ. The drugs violence nexus: A tripartite conceptual framework. Drug Issues 1985; 15:493–506.
41. Klebba AJ. Homicide trends in the United States, 1900–1974. Public Health Rep 1974; 90:195–204.
42. Cook TD, Kendzierski DA, Thomas SV. The implicit assumptions of television research: An analysis of the 1982 NIMH report on television and behavior. Public Opinion Quarterly 1983; 47:161–201.
43. Collins J. Drinking and crime. New York: Guilford Press, 1981.
44. Zahn MA, Snodgrass G. Drug use and the structure of homicide in two US cities. In: Flynn EE, Conrad JP, eds. The new and the old criminology. New York: Praeger Press, 1978.
45. Zimring FE. Determinants of the death rate from robbery: A Detroit time study. In: Rose HM, ed. Lethal aspects of urban violence. Lexington, MA: Lexington Books, 1979: 31–50.
46. Block R. Violent crime. Lexington, MA: Lexington Books, 1977.

47. Cook PJ, ed. The effect of gun availability on violent crime patterns: Gun control. Ann Am Acad Political and Soc Sci 1981; 455.
48. Cook PJ. The influence of gun availability on violent crime patterns. In: Tomy M, Morris N, eds. Crime and justice, an annual review of research, Vol. 4. Chicago: University of Chicago Press, 1983.
49. Fox JA. An econometric analysis of crime data (dissertation). University of Pennsylvania, 1976.
50. Gelles RJ. Child abuse as a psychopathology: A sociological critique and reformulation. Am J Orthopsychiatry 1973; 43:611–621.
51. Erlanger H. The empirical status of the subculture of violence thesis. Soc Problems 1974; 22:280–291.
52. Robin GD. Justifiable homicide by police officers. J Crim Law, Criminol and Police Sci 1970; 8:48–56.
53. Lundsgaarde HP. Murder in space city. New York: Oxford University Press, 1977.
54. Shichor D, Decker DL, O'Brien RM. Population density and criminal victimization—some unexpected findings in central cities. Criminology 1979; 17:184–193.
55. Curtis LA. Criminal violence—national patterns and behavior. Lexington, MA: Lexington Books, 1974.
56. Silberman CE. Criminal violence and criminal justice. New York: Vintage Books, 1978.
57. Greenwood PW. The violent offender in the criminal justice system. In: Wolfgang M, Weiner NA, eds. Criminal violence. Beverly Hills: Sage, 1982: 320–346.
58. Smith ME, Thompson JW. Employment, youth and violent crime. In: Feinberg KR, ed. Violent crime in America. Washington, DC: National Policy Exchange, 1983.
59. World Health Organization. World Health Stat Annuls. Geneva: WHO, 1986, 1987, 1988.
60. Williams KR. Economic sources of homicide; reestimating the effects of poverty and inequality. Am Soc Rev, April 1984; 49:283–289.
61. Centerwall BS. Race, socioeconomic status and domestic homicide, Atlanta, 1971–72. Am J Public Health 1984; 74(8):813–815.
62. Smith J, Mercy J, Rosenberg M. Comparison of homicides among Anglos and Hispanics in five southwestern states. Presented at U.S.-Mexico Border Health Association Meeting, Hermosillo, Mexico, April 10, 1984.
63. US Dept. of Justice. Crime in the United States, 1986. Washington, DC: US Dept. of Justice, 1987.
64. US Dept. of Justice, Bureau of Justice Statistics. Violent crime by strangers and nonstrangers: Bureau of Justice Statistics special report. Washington, DC: Bureau of Justice Statistics, US Dept. of Justice. (NCJ-103702), 1987.
65. Straus MA, Gelles JR, Steinmetz SK. Behind closed doors: Violence in the American family. New York: Anchor Press/Doubleday, 1980.
66. Stark E, Flitcraft A, Zukcerman D, et al. Wife abuse in the medical settings: An introduction for health personnel. Washington, DC: Office of Domestic Violence, 1981 (Monograph No. 7).
67. Eth S, Pynoos RS. Bearing witness: A model of research and intervention. Presented at American Psychiatric Association, May 10, 1984, Anaheim, CA.
68. Berk S, Loseke D. "Handling" family violence: the situated determinants of police arrest in domestic disturbances. Law and Society Rev 1980; 15(2):317–346.

69. Attorney General's Task Force on Family Violence. Final report, Washington, DC, September 1984.
70. National Committee for Injury Prevention and Control. Injury prevention: Meeting the challenge. New York: Oxford University Press, 1989.
71. Prothrow-Stith D. Primary prevention of homicide: Preliminary report on a demonstration project investigating the value of health education in the high school on anger and violence. Presentation at NASW-NIMH workshop on prevention of black homicide, Washington, DC, June 1984.
72. Prothrow-Stith D. Violence prevention curriculum for adolescents. Newton, MA: Education Development Center, 1987.
73. Ross CH, Zigler E. An agenda for action. In: Gerbna G, Ross CJ, Zigler E, eds. Child abuse: An agenda for action. New York: Oxford University Press, 1980: 293–304.
74. Zigler E. Controlling child abuse in America: An effort doomed to failure? In: Bourne R, Newberger EH, eds. Critical perspectives on child abuse. Lexington, MA: Lexington Books, 1979: 171–213.
75. Garbarino J. The human ecology of child maltreatment. J Mar and the Family 1977; 39:412–427.
76. Saltzman LE, Mercy JA, Rosenberg ML, et al. Magnitude and patterns of family and intimate assault in Atlanta, Georgia, 1984. Violence and Victims 1990; 5(1):3–17.
77. Blumstein A, Cohen J, Nagen D, eds. Deterrence and incapacitation: Estimating the effects of criminal sanctions on crime rates. Washington, DC: National Academy of Sciences, 1978.
78. Straus MA. Ordinary violence, child abuse, and wife beating: What do they have in common. In: Finkelhor D, Gelles R, Hotaling G, Straus M, eds. The dark side of families: Current family violence research. Beverly Hills: Sage, 1983: 213–234.
79. Greenwood PW. The violent offender in the criminal justice system. In: Wolfgang M, Weiner NA, eds. Criminal violence. Beverly Hills: Sage, 1982: 320–346.
80. Mercy JA, Houk VN. Firearm injuries: A call for science. N Eng J Med 1988; 319(19):1283–1285.
81. Wintemute GJ. Firearms as a cause of death in the United States, 1920–1982. J of Trauma 1987; 27:532–536.
82. Jagger J, Dietz PE. Death and injury by firearms: Who cares? JAMA 1986; 255:3143–3144.
83. Geisel MS, Roll R, Weltich RS Jr. The effectiveness of state and local regulation of handguns: A statistical analysis. Duke Law J 1969: 647–676.

3

Child Abuse

ELI H. NEWBERGER

Despite increasing public awareness, both clinical practice and social policy are constrained by substantial deficits in the knowledge base on child abuse and by gaps in the application of research findings to its prevention and treatment. Newer research demonstrates, for example, that psychopathology is not more prevalent in families where abuse is documented than in the general population, but the focus of clinical protective work remains primarily psychotherapeutic; and talking to an individual parent with a view to changing the parent's behavior remains the paradigm of clinical practice. Clinicians who work with families identified as having abused their children may find it difficult to conceptualize etiology and treatment of problems outside the biomedical, symptom-oriented approach to which their practice and training are oriented.

Definitions of child abuse have broadened significantly in the last two decades, expanding from an initial focus on injuries inflicted by caregivers to include the categories of neglect, sexual victimization of children inside and out of the home, and denial of necessary life support to severely handicapped infants. These increasingly broad definitions have brought into the child welfare system an increasing number of case reports, but resources have not grown commensurately. Inadequate numbers of trained personnel within and without the formal child protection system limit the effectiveness of current intervention programs.

Every human organ system can be affected by the symptoms of child abuse, and both the physical and psychological implications for child and adult development appear to be grave. Yet insufficient study has been made of the relationships between different kinds of abuse and different outcomes, thus limiting substantially the development of programs and policies.

Prevention appears to hold promise for reducing the prevalence and impact of child abuse, and the principal preventive initiatives can be derived from specific theories of causality. In addition to making a commitment toward prevention, further efforts should be made to understand the etiology and epidemiology of child abuse and the effectiveness of interventions.

STATEMENT OF THE PROBLEM

The commonsense meaning of the term "child abuse" is a situation where a caregiver, generally a parent, sets out in a systematic way to harm a defenseless child. This is the notion of the problem in most medical settings, deriving from the relatively recent "discovery" by the medical profession of an age-old phenomenon. Attention was drawn to the problem in 1962 by Professor C. Henry Kempe and his associates in an influential article in the *Journal of the American Medical Association* (JAMA), entitled "The Battered Child Syndrome" (1). This study prompted an outpouring of editorial concern in professional and lay media. It was the stimulus for the drafting by the Children's Bureau, the lead agency for children in the federal government, of a model child abuse reporting statute. Child abuse came to be defined in the state reporting laws as injuries inflicted by caregivers. These, it was widely held, could be diagnosed by physicians and medical institutions. And if physicians could be required to report child abuse cases to public agencies, principally to welfare departments, a response competent to assure the safety of the children would logically ensue (2,3).

The year 1962 was a time of great public concern for the rights of disadvantaged citizens in the United States. The success of the civil rights movement in bringing to public attention the suffering of black Americans was reflected in the passage by Congress and state legislatures of laws to open opportunities to vote, to go to school, and to live without fear of violent reprisal for overstepping the codes of segregation. Also prevailing at this time was a sense of the role and responsibility of government in helping disadvantaged citizens, including children. The five years subsequent to the publication of "The Battered Child Syndrome" also saw the advent of several major new programs to benefit children: regional centers for retarded children, stimulated by President John F. Kennedy's own concern for his sister; Project Headstart, which provided child care and related health and family services for disadvantaged children; and Medicaid, a program to provide payment for health services to indigent people, with a special provision for children whose families are dependent on public welfare. This provision stipulated that these children were all to be given early and periodic screening, diagnosis, and treatment services ("EPSDT") for conditions that might limit their health or development.

The time was ripe for the medical discovery of child abuse, and the title of the Kempe article in JAMA telegraphed a vivid sense of its meaning and of the professions' and agencies' roles: it was for physicians to make the "diagnosis," and, as formalized in the child abuse reporting statutes, it was the responsibility of the agencies mandated to receive the reports to provide the "treatment." But the article's perpetrator-victim model of etiology and the notion of a *syndrome* of physical examination findings in the child and psychopathology in the caregiver led to several problematic consequences.

These persist to the present day. Physicians confuse the ethics of making a diagnosis and giving care with the functions of investigation (to find out who did what to whom and how); a mythology persists that all adults who harm children in their care are mentally ill; and agencies that receive the reports maintain a conflicted sense of responsibility. Although the legal mandate may be to offer services to protect the children and help their families, the persistence of the perpetrator-victim model substantially inhibits the range of perceived diagnostic and therapeutic possibilities in these agencies; in the face of enormous caseloads and shortened resources, whether or not to separate a child from his or her parents' care becomes the informing question of practice, and punishment may be meted out in the guise of help (4).

The public and professional activism of the 1960s stimulated studies of the child abuse phenomenon, and these studies affected the efforts during the early 1970s to revise the laws mandating the reporting of child abuse. Parents of abused children were acknowledged to be people who could be helped, and child abuse came to be seen as a form of human trouble not unrelated to other family disturbances, with implications for the health and welfare of children. This humane perspective was reflected in the title of an influential book edited by Professor Kempe and his colleague, pediatrician Ray Helfer, *Helping the Battered Child and His Family* (5).

In this view, government's role was to provide timely help to troubled families whose children might bear physical and behavioral symptoms that could be acknowledged not only by doctors, but by other observers as well. A new model child abuse reporting law was promulgated by the Children's Bureau of the U.S. Department of Health, Education, and Welfare, the agency that was given the responsibility to house the National Center on Child Abuse and Neglect. This center was created by Public Law 93-247 and signed into law by President Richard M. Nixon early in 1973.

This draft statute proposed broadening the definition of child abuse to include neglect, emotional injury, parental deprivation of medical care, and factors injurious to a child's moral development. It lengthened the list of professionals required by law to make child abuse case reports to include virtually anyone responsible for the care of children. The committee that drafted the model statute was cautioned by the federal officials of the sponsoring agency against including any language that might link the reporting process to budgeting for services. Although a dramatic increase in reports was foreseen, the assumption was that the good consciences of the state legislators would contend with the cost implications of the statutes (6). Further, the states were given an important incentive by the National Center to bring their laws into conformity with the new model reporting statute: unless their statutes conformed, they would not be eligible for their share of the federal monies that P.L. 93-247 stipulated should go for improving state services.

The resulting broadening of the public definitions, associated with public awareness campaigns by the National Center and by the private National Committee for the Prevention of Child Abuse, reflected the understanding of child abuse held by professionals working in the field as well as much of the general public, that "child abuse" was not restricted to parents setting out to destroy their defenseless offspring.

In retrospect, one unforeseen consequence of that effort was a changing sense of the government's responsibility for children and families in trouble. States such as Florida, which introduced the new reporting legislation with public service announcements in the major electronic media, were promptly deluged with more reports than could be managed by the limited numbers of child welfare personnel (7). A subsequent study of a random sample of Florida child abuse case reports was stimulated in part by press inquiries into reinjuries and deaths associated with superficial screenings of reports. At this screening stage, reports were either "screened in" as "valid" and referred to a caseworker for investigation, or "screened out" as "invalid" and no investigation pursued. This study showed that it was the professional status of the reporter and not the contents of the report on the child that determined whether a report would be screened in as valid (8). Reports from physicians were far more frequently screened in than those, for example, from child care workers.

Child welfare agencies are now overburdened in every state. The expanded definition of child abuse has led to another paradoxical and troubling issue at a time when resources to support families are in increasingly short supply. In many jurisdictions, the only way to get publicly funded child care or residential psychiatric treatment services is to file a child abuse case report, because these services are no longer available as child welfare services *per se*. As a result, many professionals face the dilemma that in order to help a family, they may have to condemn the parents as "bad" by reporting them as child abusers. This notion of a professional duty to protect child victims from their bad and abusive parents is reflected in the new name for these services: child welfare services have become child protection services in most states. The submission by the Attorney General's Task Force on Family Violence of a report urging an increased use of criminal prosecution in all such cases indicates a strong dissatisfaction with the failures of child protection services (9).

In the 1985 reauthorization of the National Center on Child Abuse and Neglect, child abuse was conceived still more broadly to include situations where handicapped infants may be denied medical care necessary to assure their survival. The regulations promulgated by the Children's Bureau required states to set up specialized units within their protective service programs to investigate and pursue reports of such denials of care. These stimulated a huge amount of correspondence, including protests from the principal associations of medical specialists, including the American

Academy of Pediatrics (10). They objected strenuously to this intrusion by the government into the judgments of practice.

The mounting public awareness of child sexual victimization and the highly publicized cases of sexual abuse of children in day care centers have led to yet another initiative to expand the concept of child abuse and the role of child protection agencies. Federal regulations (1985) require the investigation by child protection agencies of reports of abuse in institutional settings such as day care centers (11).

The definition of what constitutes a "case" of child abuse has been changed dramatically in the last quarter-century. Although to many if not most medical professionals, the "battered child syndrome" model appears to prevail, other professions, caregiving institutions, and agencies of government have defined the problem more expansively. But the notion of fault, whether it be the caregiver's active or passive hurting or denying necessary care to the child, remains implicit in the definitions, narrow or broad. This leads to a practice of making burdensome judgments and involving in children's and families' lives agencies that are not always seen as helpful and in many cases may be seen by them and by others as inept, intrusive, hurtful, and punitive. The physician is trained to avoid making value judgments about the people he or she serves, to hold confidential information given in the setting of practice, and to keep in mind two universal doctrines of good practice. The doctrine of *informed consent* obliges the physician to make known any risks or adverse outcomes that might result from the physician's work, and indeed not to proceed with any interventions that might carry the possibility of harm without the patient's explicit agreement. The *Hippocratic axiom* states, first of all, do no harm. Both of these ethical doctrines are challenged in nearly every aspect of conforming to the requirements of the reporting statutes. For many doctors, the decision *not* to report a case of child abuse, however child abuse might be conceived, is taken with great seriousness and attention to the high principles of ethical care.

The problem, then, is not simply a set of injuries that parents may inflict through passive or active means on their children. The conception of child abuse is affected importantly by the political and social meaning of the protection of children in the United States at the end of the twentieth century. Child protection, and by inference child abuse, has become a vehicle to influence medical practice, for example, to assure the provision of life support to severely handicapped newborns; it has become the device to justify the distribution of scarce family support resources at a time when it is no longer possible to make them available on the basis of need alone; and it is proposed as a mechanism to police proliferating child care institutions as more and more women enter the workforce and leave their children in these settings.

The picture of child abuse seen in medical practice depends on how the problem is understood. In the words of the radiologists, "You see what you look for, and you look for what you know." For practitioners oriented to a perpetrator-victim model, the field of vision may be restricted to such major findings as fractures, bruises to portions of the body that would not ordinarily occur in play (bruises not over bony prominences and conforming to the shapes of sticks, looped electric cords, teeth, and fingers will generally raise suspicion), scalds (especially in glove or stocking distributions), collections of blood around, above, or beneath the dense lining of the brain (which may be due to direct trauma or to violent shaking), poisonings, lacerations, and contusions to internal organs. These injuries evoke greater concern when children are younger and when different forms of trauma occur simultaneously or over time (12).

A more embracing medical concept of child abuse, which proposes to go beyond the perpetrator-victim model and to foster a practice in which the process of diagnosis is not jeopardized by the need to assign blame, draws attention to the relationships among the "pediatric social illnesses," unintentional injuries, poisonings, and the condition known as "failure to thrive," where children fail to gain weight and length at adequate rates, but where no definable illness can be found to explain the growth failure (13,14). The child's physical symptoms are understood in an ecologic framework that includes these interacting elements: the given child's unique developmental qualities and risk; the parents' adaptation to the child's caregiving needs, and particularly their capacities to nurture and to protect the child from harm; the psychological attributes of the family, both with respect to the individual's vulnerabilities and strengths and to their relationships with a family system; the realities and exigencies of the nurturing or holding environment, including hazards, the perceived quality of the neighborhood, and the family's connections to or isolation from kin and other supports; and the favorable and unfavorable qualities of professional personnel, service programs, and institutions with which they may have contact.

Practice should focus more on family strengths and on prevention rather than on perceived pathologies to be treated by health care professionals. This may necessitate abandoning the highly pejorative characterizations of family life suggested by the name "child abuse." Ultimately as well, the notions of "reporting" a family for treatment by a state agency may give way to a more generous and humane sense of how a child's symptoms reflect particular family relationships and caregiving practices (15). Given the present trend toward criminalization of family disturbances in the United States, there is concern that the promise of help in the child abuse reporting statutes may turn out to be an empty promise for many children.

Recent attention has also been drawn to two entities of particular concern to physicians and other medical workers, the "Munchausen syndrome by proxy" and the problem of sexual victimization of children by professionals, including physicians (16–20). Munchausen syndrome has been used to describe the adult patient who falsifies medical history and physical examination findings. In its pediatric manifestation, it is the parent (the "designated culprit of deceit," in the uncharitable words of an article in *Pediatrics*, the official journal of the American Academy of Pediatrics [21]) who is posited to make the child ill, presumably to draw attention to his or her problems.

Children are described in the case reports who have had their skin scratched with needles to give the impression of a bleeding disorder, who have been given injections of fecal matter to produce bizarre patterns of fever, and who have been subjected repeatedly to intrusive diagnostic procedures. These cases stimulate many conflicts for physicians because the childrens' mothers often seem like ideal parents who are especially grateful for the doctor's interest and care, and because it is often more convenient to perform diagnostic studies than it is to question the validity of the proffered history. Many of the mothers have worked as nurses or nursing aides or cared for chronically ill relatives. The medical office is the favored entry point for these patients.

The victimization of children by nonparental caretakers is a subject of increasing concern, perhaps as a consequence of the broad attention given to child sexual abuse in day care centers. In some cases, especially when several staff members are involved, this may reflect the larger, linked problems of pedophilia, child pornography, and sex rings (22,23). Many pedophiles are oriented to children in a particular age bracket and sex. They may memorialize their experiences in photographs, journals, letters, and videotapes in order to maintain stimuli for fantasy as the children grow out of the preferred ages. Sex rings involve adults with similar orientations who may exploit large numbers of children by sexual acts and by the trading and selling of mementos.

The association between child abuse and other forms of family violence has been highlighted by tragedies, such as the murder of Lisa Steinberg in New York City, which drew attention to the connection between the problems of battered women and child abuse (24). There also appears to be an important link with the family issues associated with homelessness (25).

DATA SOURCES

There are few data sources on child abuse that permit useful inferences to be drawn on prevalence, incidence, risk factors, outcomes, and the effectiveness of interventions. This is a consequence of the selective nature of case ascertainment for clinical research, the limitations of study design in nearly every clinical study, and of a reluctance in the formation of national policy on child abuse to make use of standard methods of measurement and program evaluation.

Clinical studies are rarely controlled and thus are nearly entirely confounded by socioeconomic class and age artifacts. Few samples are ascertained from any but institutional settings. The generalizability of most of the clinical reports is severely restricted (26).

The major data sets on child abuse, all established with the support of federal government grants, give some useful estimates of reported prevalence, and four studies demonstrate the utility of methodologies that do not rely on case reports. The first major data set was established by Professor

David Gil of Brandeis University and is the first systematic treatment of child abuse case reports to agencies mandated by the initial wave of reporting statutes in the early and middle 1960s (27). Gil also purchased under his contract with the Children's Bureau several questions on a public opinion poll conducted by the National Opinion Research Center at the University of Chicago.

Respondents in a national probability sample (i.e., representative of the major demographic attributes of the national population) were asked, for example, whether they personally knew of a case of child abuse; from this Gil extrapolated an incidence estimate of between two and a half million cases per year. Gil's analysis of 1967 and 1968 case reports serves as the benchmark study of its kind. The study's conclusion that poverty is the principal determinant of abuse has been criticized on the grounds that the demographic attributes of the reported cases reflect the class and other biases of the reporting process. The Gil data were used productively by Light, who explored the possible utility of parent education and risk-screening policies (28).

The American Humane Association contracts with the Children's Bureau to compile official reports of child abuse and neglect, but for several reasons these annual compilations are of less value than the original study performed by Gil. The absence of standardized definitions, dependence on the individual states' data aggregation methods, and inability to gauge the meaning of the case reports in reference to any sampling methodology means that these reports describe mainly who it is who gets into the child protection system bearing the tag of abuse or neglect. These reports present a confusing picture with regard to time trends, for example, as state statutes have broadened the definitions of reportable conditions and, in the face of budgetary retrenchments for other child welfare services, many cases flow into the system because a child abuse case report is the only device available to attract publicly funded services.

Notwithstanding these limitations, the AHA data give a lively impression of the number and nature of "caught" cases and a sense of how the child abuse problem has grown. Where in 1967 and 1968, Gil documented only 6,000 to 7,000 case reports a year, the 1986 AHA survey of state reports yielded an estimated prevalence of 1,928,000 abused children (29). As with the Gil data, most of the reports were on behalf of children in indigent families, reflecting in part the bias of ascertainment that favors poor children to be reported to agencies of the state that are seen as poor people's agencies. AHA data also document an increasing number of cases of child sexual victimization, perhaps in response to elevated public and professional awareness generated by extensive media attention to sexual abuse. These increased levels of reporting may also reflect the trends in divorce and the improvised child care arrangements of single working mothers that may place their children at risk of sexual victimization by boyfriends, relatives, or other caregivers out of the parental home.

Unfortunately, an effort has never been made to assemble and to integrate the case report data with a survey of the population in such a way as to permit an estimate of the true prevalence of child abuse, neglect, and sexual victimization. Nor has there been an analysis of the year-to-year case report data with information collected by the Bureau of the Census and other agencies on the changes in the structure of the American family, especially with regard to divorce, women in the workforce (1985 data suggest that over half the women with preschool children work full time [30]), and child-care arrangements. Neither have the data been compared with the Uniform Crime Reports of the Department of Justice, nor injury or hospital data collected by the National Center for Health Statistics and other units of the U.S. Public Health Service.

Representative sampling methodologies have been used to estimate the incidence and prevalence of child abuse. Murray Straus and his associates have pioneered the use of direct interview methods in which people are asked about their practices and experiences. Straus's collaboration with Richard Gelles and Suzanne Steinmetz produced the first national survey of family violence. This survey utilized a scale to measure the techniques family members used to resolve conflicts among themselves; in turn, this scale provided the entry point for a series of questions about violent practices (31).

Using a national sample of families with two adults and at least one child between three and seventeen years of age, Straus and his colleagues produced the first systematic and reliable projections of the frequency of particular incidents of violence, such as using or threatening to use a knife or a gun in resolving conflict with another specific family member in the last year or ever. Their study also yielded some of the first family-level insights into the meaning of violence. For example, women who were victims of severe violence at the hands of their spouses were 150 percent more likely to use severe violence in resolving conflicts with their children. Their sample, however, was not representative of American families with children. Because of the investigators' interest in acts of violence between adults and among children and adults, infants were not represented, and neglect or sexual victimization was not explored. The study yielded a prevalence estimate suggesting that in 1975 there were 1.4 million children ages three to seventeen years who had been abused.

Gelles and Straus have recently reported the findings of a second national family violence survey, which yielded a much lower prevalence estimate. The extent to which nonscientific issues may affect public discourse on the prevalence and incidence of child abuse is described in their book-length report of the survey:

The shock we felt when we first examined our data was echoed when we presented the results at professional meetings. The data on violence toward children were presented at the Seventh National Conference on Child Abuse and Neglect, which was sponsored by the National Center on Child Abuse and Neglect and the National Committee for Prevention of Child Abuse. In preparing for the conference, the National Committee had set an almost unprecedented goal by calling for the reduction of child abuse by 20% by 1990. Hundreds of conferees wore buttons that said *20% by 1990* while we presented data that reported that the rate of severe violence had already dropped by 47%. Not surprisingly, our results were received with great skepticism (32, p. 109).

Gelles and Straus review the principal methodological artifacts that may have led to an underestimate of prevalence: 1975 data were collected using in-person interviews; 1985 interviews were conducted over the telephone. Families without telephones were not studied, thus excluding 5% of the population, a group more likely to experience social isolation and economic adversity. Respondents were perhaps less willing to report family violence in 1985 than they were in 1975. The authors of the study assert their belief, however, that there has been a decline in the rates of violence toward children and, to a lesser extent, women (32, p. 111).

A so-called national incidence study of child abuse and neglect was funded by the Children's Bureau in response to a congressional mandate under the terms of the reauthorization of the National Center on Child Abuse and Neglect. A study was designed to delineate the dimensions of the "iceberg" of child abuse, only the tip of which was believed to show in child abuse case reports. Levels of visibility of child abuse were postulated and then plumbed by gathering data from child protective agencies (the figurative tip) and such other sources as hospitals, police departments, and mental health agencies (33). Systematic definitions were promulgated, and cases from the various reporting sources were ascertained by telephone or by form. Data from the various sources were then aggregated. A weighting system was devised to generalize to the national experience. For the 26-county sample, 17,645 cases of child abuse and neglect came to attention between May 1, 1979, and April 30, 1980; it was projected that nationwide 1,151,600 cases were suspected by professionals. Of these projected cases, 562,000 were considered as likely to meet the study's criteria, i.e., represented true cases of child abuse and neglect.

The method of study has been criticized discerningly by Finkelhor and Hotaling. They noted that child sexual victimization was rarely reported at the time of the incidence study. Because 95 percent of these cases came to the study's attention through child protection or other investigatory agencies (for example, the police), there were likely to have been a far greater number of sexual abuse cases than the study measured (34).

Sexual victimization prevalence and the characteristics of victims and their families have been studied using survey methodology by Finkelhor and his coworkers (35–37). The findings suggest a far greater frequency than the case reporting compilations would suggest, with prevalence estimates between 8 percent and 62 percent of women, and 5 percent and 30 percent of men, depending on the breadth of definition, the ages surveyed, and the sampling methods.

The first national incidence study data are now available for others' use and are especially useful for studies of agency practice, for example, with regard to the case attributes that drive the reporting practices of hospitals, especially class and race (38).

A second national incidence study employed a similar methodology and the same contractor (Westat, Inc.) (39). The data for 1986 are presented in the recently published report, along with perceived changes since the earlier study. The estimated 1986 national incidence of abuse and neglect was 1,584,700. There was a 74 percent increase in the incidence of abuse (to 657,000 cases), within which there was an increase of 58 percent for child physical abuse (to 358,300 cases) and over 300 percent for child sexual abuse (to 155,900 cases). No changes were noted in the incidence of emotional abuse or neglect. Physical abuse was the most frequent type of abuse identified in the study, followed by emotional abuse and by sexual abuse, with respective incidence rate estimates of 5.7, 3.4,and 2.5 cases per thousand children. With regard to the shape of the child abuse "iceberg," there were no changes in the proportion of cases that were reported to state child protection agencies, but more stringent screening standards by these agencies indicate "that some of the children who would, in the past, have had their cases substantiated (and possibly received services as a result) are now excluded as unfounded" (39, p. xxv).

Data sources on child abuse are constrained by inconsistent definitions, a relentless focus on the study of reported or "caught" cases, confounding by social class and other uncontrolled attributes, inadequate generalizability of the findings, the theoretical and disciplinary biases of funding agencies and scholars, and by an absence of linkage between demonstration programs, research funding, and efforts to make sense of the findings for program development and public policy.

The measurement and analysis of the prevalence and incidence of the many problems now identified under the rubric of "child abuse" would seem to require consistent attention to epidemiologic concepts and methods, regular and systematic review of measurement alternatives and their relationships to the mechanisms for official case identification and reporting, and an orientation to current theory and knowledge of etiology and prevention. By contrast, the present approach to this vital public health function is to assign the tasks of measurement on an occasional basis to contractors who submit bids for specified pieces of work. A specific governmental unit, charged with the responsibility for assessing the magnitude and severity of child abuse, might be better able to attend appropriately to the issues of technique, as the National Center on Child Abuse and Neglect with its overburdened staff and lack of epidemiologic expertise cannot do. This might assure the availability of data and reasoned interpretation at a level of quality commensurate with the seriousness of the problem.

CAUSES AND RISK FACTORS

Initial efforts to understand child abuse focused on the psychological problems of the parents of the victims. The influential study by Steele and
Pollock pointed to abusing parents' distorted expectations of their children,
frustrated dependency needs, personal isolation, and histories of having
themselves been abused as children (40). Helfer has suggested that risk to a
child for abuse may be understood as having three fundamental dimensions:
a child with qualities that are provocative; a parent with the psychological
predisposition; and a stressful event that triggers a violent reaction (41). In
addition to causes originating in the family, social and cultural factors have
also been described, dispelling the widely held myth that it is exclusively
individual deviant behavior that culminates in child abuse (42–45).

The psychoanalytic approach posits that unconscious parental drives and
conflicts determine the behavior we characterize as abuse (40,46). This
theory organizes the knowledge gathered by many psychologically minded
clinicians, and, indeed, informed Kempe's perceptions of the parents of the
victims of the "battered child syndrome." The abusive caregiver was characterized in that work as the "psychopathological member of the family."

Social learning theory suggests that child abuse is learned behavior and
that individuals who have experienced violent and abusive childhoods are
more likely to grow up to become child and spouse abusers than individuals
who experienced little or no violence in their childhood years (47). Violence
in one's family of origin is seen as predictive of violence in one's family of
procreation.

Environmental stress theory posits that the child abuse results from social
and environmental stress. Stressful life conditions and events, including
poverty, unemployment, social isolation, inadequate housing, and a violent
social milieu are prominent factors considered with this theoretical orientation (48). This perspective suggests that factors in the context of family life
that are felt as overwhelmingly stressful facilitate the expression of violence
or interfere with a parent's ability to care for his or her children.

Cognitive-developmental theory proposes that child abuse reflects an
immature parental understanding of the child and of the parental role (49).
Four levels of parental thinking about children and the parent-child relationships have been described, some of which are associated with child
abuse, especially when coupled with family stresses.

Labeling theory presumes social inequality and suggests that the interests
of dominant power groups are served by defining as deviant a class of
socially marginal individuals (the "child abusers") whose individual problems become the proper concerns of the helping professionals (50).

Each of the above theories can be described as a unitary theory since each
offers an explanation of child abuse from a single point of view. Each theory
has power and adherents because it explains some part of the data, but each
also has clear limitations. Psychoanalytic explanations, for example, have

guided much of the work in this field, but when abusive parents have been studied, only one parent in ten has been found to have a definable psychiatric condition, a figure comparable to the rest of the population (51). Further, child abuse has been found to be associated with several personality types, and no particular psychiatric diagnosis can predict abuse (52).

Other unitary theories share comparable limitations. For example, environmental stress theory does not take into account intraindividual and interindividual sources of strength and weakness that may render families more or less vulnerable to environmental experiences and conditions. Nor do they account for child abuse in seemingly affluent homes. And labeling theory, although helpful in pointing out pervasive biases with respect to who gets identified and reported as abusive, is of scant help in the emergency room when addressing the needs of a family whose child has cigarette burns on its body.

Professionals and researchers are becoming more alert to the conceptual underpinnings of empirical research on child abuse and critically evaluating the utility of unitary theories of etiology, and, as a result, they are integrating the more helpful parts of these theories into interactive, multicausal theories. These multicausal theories seek to understand how aspects of an individual's personality or environment may interact with his or her particular experience. Are particular personality types more susceptible to the stresses of certain kinds of environmental experiences? Are there features of the social environment, or ways of understanding a child, that enable families to cope with stress without resorting to violence?

Several studies have attempted to integrate causal factors for child abuse from multiple levels: individual, family, and society (53–56). At the individual level, an important and consistent finding is the prevalence of acute or chronic illness in victims of child abuse (57–60). This causal association has systematically been neglected in child protection agency practice, because case workers have limited and fixed notions of the etiology of child abuse and because service agencies are already overburdened and do not have the requisite resources for medical diagnosis and treatment. When North Carolina and Florida made medical consultation available to social workers in child protection agencies, medical antecedents and concomitants of child abuse became increasingly acknowledged (61–62).

Certain individual and family factors that have been accepted as "causes" of child abuse must now be contemplated with skepticism. Among these are low birth weight of the infant, young maternal age, and inadequate mother-infant "bond formation" (63–64).

Gelles has documented a pervasive, uncritical acceptance by professionals of empirical assertions about child abuse (65). He draws on the "woozle" metaphor from *Winnie the Pooh*, in which two characters stalk an imaginary beast around a tree, tracking one another's footprints. Many "woozles" are found in the literature on child abuse: simple, empirical results or statements, reiterated by many authors, gain the status of axioms or laws, even though the findings may be in error. Clinical practice based on oft-repeated but essentially erroneous findings may be ineffective or even harmful. A familiar example to those who work in the clinical environment is the tidy home woozle. A case report of inflicted injury is made, and the social worker who visits the family notes that the house is clean and orderly. Referring to page 55 of the Massachusetts 1985 "Reference Guide for Child Abuse and Neglect Investigations," he or she will note under Condition of the Home the following: "An example of a home which poses a *low* risk to a child is one which is clean, with no apparent safety hazards such as exposed wiring or rodent infestation, and structurally sound" (66). The focus of child protection services on poor families has led to a sense of connection between a home in poor repair and a child in danger, although the fact that a home is neat may bear no relationship to a child's risk of abuse. A social worker using the cited reference guide may wrongly conclude that the risk of reinjury to the child is small.

Academic behavioral and social science research has not, in general, produced results that are applicable in clinical settings. Much survey research, for example, applies a factor-by-factor approach in attempting to statistically explain the child abuse phenomenon. Both the method of study and the format in which the results are reported may ignore the complexity of individual cases—each of which involves interactions among personal history, general social context, and immediate situational factors. The conclusions drawn from statistical analysis of large sample surveys, when they are communicated to clinicians, may be swallowed eagerly as tools for simple clinical decision making or dismissed as glib and useless. Other social science theories such as social exchange theory may take into account the complexity of individual interaction with families, but their relevance to clinical application may not be immediately apparent; the usual focus of the academic researcher is on the formulation of universal rules ("nomothetic" principles) that govern behavior, whereas the clinician's concern is with executing particular treatment programs appropriate to individual cases.

Despite such differences between clinical practice and academic research, there are important points of fruitful interchange and shared development. Structural family therapy, with its emphasis on the family as a system of independent actors, contains assumptions similar to those of social exchange theory, which emphasizes interaction, coalition formation, and the exchange of rewards and punishments. Discussions between academic researchers and clinicians permit cross-fertilization between such perspectives.

Clinicians from various fields of practice and researchers from different disciplines can benefit from working together on the study of treatment of child abuse. Such cooperation should help develop a taxonomy of violent acts, a more reliable body of etiologic explanations, indications for different therapeutic interventions, effective prevention programs based on understandings of etiology, and relevant family policies. Unless and until such cooperation and a shared sense of mission can develop, knowledge of the causes and risks associated with child abuse will be restricted.

OUTCOMES

Child abuse is costly in both human and fiscal terms, but neither the medical nor the psychological sequelae have been studied sufficiently well to allow a conclusive assessment of their costs. This is partly a consequence of policies regarding the funding of research. The principal federal agency responsible for research on child health, the National Institute of Child Health and Human Development in the National Institutes of Health, has taken the position since the early 1970s that it will not support studies of child abuse; the National Center on Child Abuse and Neglect, after funding three short-term studies of the impact of child physical abuse, announced in its July 1985 priority statement additional support for studies of the impact of child sexual victimization. These projects were not to exceed three years.

The documented medical consequences of child abuse include injuries inflicted on every organ system, not infrequently causing chronic impairment (67). Injuries to the central nervous system from direct trauma or shaking appear to be responsible for many cases of cerebral palsy and profound neurologic impairment (68). The costs of treatment and of lost productivity have not been studied.

Homicide, one of the five leading causes of death for children between the ages of 1 and 18 years, is another outcome of child abuse. Homicides involving infants are not always accurately classified and are probably underreported (69,70). The impact of homicide is more fully appreciated when one considers the number of years of potential life lost and lost productivity; the 501 child homicides committed in 1980 account for 93,000 years of potential life lost (71).

Child sexual victimization culminated in the transmission of venereal disease in 13 percent of the 409 children in one study, and included gonorrhea, syphilis, condyloma acuminata, and trichomoniasis (72). Herpes genitalis and chlamydia are also documented sequelae of child sexual abuse (73).

The long-term psychological effects of child abuse have been described in various case compilations, but varying definitions of abuse, problematic investigative methodologies, and differences in outcome criteria yield a mixed impression of the impacts. In recent reviews there appears to be a consensus on a profound and serious set of effects (74–76). For child physical abuse, these include disturbances in social and emotional development, including a propensity to aggression in adolescence; violence toward intimates; language disorders; and lower performance on standardized tests of intelligence. Unfortunately, however, a prevalent sampling bias that favors the selection of impoverished children for study makes it impossible to separate the developmental attrition associated with low social class from the presumed effects of abuse (77).

McCord's 40-year follow-up of children in the Cambridge-Somerville youth study suggested insidious long-term effects of "treatment" as well as abuse and has stimulated critical discussion of classification and intervention (78–80). He found that the clinicians' characterizations of the 49 men who were said to have been abused as children carried predictive meaning (81). Abused boys were more likely than others to have been exposed to high demands for adult behavior; about half of the abused or neglected boys had subsequently been convicted for serious crimes, became alcoholic or mentally ill, or died when unusually young. They had higher rates of juvenile delinquency than those boys who were classified as having had loving parents. Although paternal alcoholism and criminal behavior were not associated with the occurrence of child abuse, they were associated with higher frequencies of later antisocial behavior. Maternal self-confidence seemed to cushion the impact of early adversity.

Although the immediate and long-term effects of child sexual victimization are the focus of much current concern, they have not been systematically studied. Such studies are needed to help develop practices and programs that could cushion the impact of child sexual victimization. From clinical case series, changes described as concomitant and subsequent to sexual abuse include hypervigilance, specific phobias, nightmares, feelings of guilt and shame, and changes in sleeping and eating patterns (82–84). Psychosomatic disorders include abdominal pain, headaches, and loss of appetite. When force is used to coerce a child into participating in sexual acts, the subsequent symptoms appear to be more severe, and the behavioral outcomes are more fully explained by analyses that simultaneously examine several variables and their interactions (85–87). Among the more important variables are the existence of antecedent behavioral problems, the family's support of the child after disclosure, the extent to which the child may have been blamed or stigmatized, and the nature and quality of the interventions on behalf of the child. So-called dissociative responses may be associated with the subsequent development of multiple personality (88,89). Additional outcomes have been reported to follow child sexual abuse, but without controlled studies it cannot be said with certainty that they were caused by the victimization.

Boys' sexual victimization may be associated with a developmental propensity to violence toward others; turning from victim to victimizer may assure the person that he is no longer vulnerable, and the sense of mastery over others may compensate for the recurrent sense of helplessness (90,91). Childhood sexual victimization appears as a frequent finding in studies of the histories and psychological characteristics of incarcerated pedophiles, rapists, and murderers (92). Women who have been sexually victimized as children appear to have an unusual frequency of depression and self-destructive behavior, as well as disturbances in adult sexual functioning and in protecting themselves from subsequent victimizing relationships (93,94).

INTERVENTIONS

For the individual practitioner, implicit in the clinical diagnosis of child abuse is a sense of parental failure. In the formulation of an intervention program, the clinician must first contend with the feelings of despair, sadness, rage, and anxiety that the case may stimulate. Many professionals and many more laypeople retain the belief that once the diagnosis of abuse is made, there is no hope for the child in his or her family. Additionally, there is often a strong impulse toward retribution against the designated perpetrator, as well as toward whomever might have been responsible for protecting the child from harm. Swift and effective punishment is now also favored by an influential report, which suggests that marital violence recidivism was reduced most effectively by the police arresting the offender (as compared to the other customary police methods of attempting to counsel both parties or sending the alleged assailant from the home for a short time) (95). This report was the basis of the recommendation for criminal process in *all* cases of family violence, child abuse included, promulgated in the Attorney General's Task Force on Family Violence.

Although child abuse may indeed be defined by many people as a crime, most social policy in the United States has inclined toward a human service model for most victims. An awkward tension now prevails between the advocates of the criminal process and the advocates of professional clinical services. Those who support the criminal process are skeptical of the utility of helping approaches and believe in the social deterrent functions of the criminal system; the advocates of professional service to children are mindful of the value of good clinical work and are concerned about the unpredictable nature of a criminal system that may itself victimize children. The paradigmatic case is that of a 12-year-old California girl whose family sought help in 1983 for an undisclosed problem of a sexual nature. The child's stepfather, a physician, was alleged in a mandated child abuse case report to have sexually abused her. The case was referred to the district attorney, who initiated a criminal action against the physician. When the girl refused to testify against her stepfather, the district attorney asked the court to find her in contempt of court. The judge ordered her held in solitary confinement until she agreed to testify. A higher court to which the matter was appealed ordered her released. The system designed to protect this child victimized her further (96).

Recently, mounting numbers of child abuse case reports have combined with local, state, and national budgetary retrenchments to seriously overburden child protection services. Efforts to shore up the protective service system have been met with resistance on the part of the politicians who are worried about the costs of meeting the needs of the numbers of children who are coming to attention through the reporting process, and on the part of the administrators who are trying to protect the integrity of their agencies from outside criticisms, however well intended.

Effective use of a tool from the civil rights movement, the class action suit, has proved successful in Massachusetts in lowering caseloads (to 18 cases per social worker), investigations (to 12 cases per social worker), and the burden of paperwork to which all welfare employees are subjected. As a result of this class action suit, training has been increased in quality and amount, and needs assessments will be performed, aggregating disparities between what children and families are perceived to need and what the Department of Social Services can provide and folding the needs into the annual budget proposal; a modern, computer-supported management information system is being set in place; medical and health needs of children in substitute care will be addressed; and recruitment and training of foster parents will be made more systematic and effective (97). Before the signing of the agreement that brought these changes into being in 1984, the case was litigated for seven years.

The decisions made by the personnel responsible for protecting children are, regrettably, often made in haste and without sufficient attention to family strengths that might be supported by homemakers, child care, parent aides, self-help groups such as Parents Anonymous, or specialized medical or psychiatric interventions. One study documented that the unavailability or cost of these supports often drives the decision to remove a child from his or her family; a strong accompanying editorial comment by a leading student of child welfare services, Professor David Fanshel of Columbia University, suggested an implicitly punitive mission of current social policies in the United States: "Given the current abandonment of federal support for social programs in the guise of block grants, the inability to show appropriate compassion for failing parents must be seen as another example of blaming the victim. There is strong indication that these parents, particularly those who are black, Hispanic, or native American, suffer from gross failure of society to adequately deliver health, mental health, and addiction services as well as suffering major deficits in income, housing, and social resources" (98,99).

Even knowledge about the family context of child abuse is too often ignored in practice. Examples are the presence of interspousal violence; the unique characteristics of a particular child; the attributes of the family and the environment, including individual roles and the family power structure; access to other people; crises in the ecologic setting (for example, with regard to housing); and the extent to which intrusions by social and health agencies may exacerbate family problems.

A doctor may suspect child abuse based on the physical examination, but if the child's mother does not appear to be mentally ill, he or she may set aside the findings and take no action, say, to report the case. A physician's practice may be constrained by popular myth (that all abused parents are mentally ill or poor or nonwhite), by past experience with protective service personnel (for whom removing a child from parental care may be the only action in the therapeutic armamentarium), by financial realities and concerns (the time spent in lengthy conversation with a family in making a case report to a protective service agency and in testifying in a custody hearing will almost certainly not be compensated), by a fear of a malpractice action deriving from the family's dissatisfaction, by class and cultural biases (a reluctance to take action to protect a child when the family is affluent or a zeal to wrest a child from the family's care when the family is poor or nonwhite), and by the emotional impact of the case. (The sadness and rage that child abuse stimulates in all of us may be intolerable to the physician, for whom an objective and dispassionate professional image may be transcendent. Faced with unpleasant feelings, it may be easier to deny the data and forget the case, in the interest of preserving emotional equilibrium.)

Interventions on behalf of victims of child abuse must attend to their needs for protection, but a widely held principle of present practice stipulates that efforts to protect a child must go hand in hand with the development of a program to help his or her family (100), including those situations where a child's future offspring need also to be considered.

An analysis of a child abuse program at one children's hospital suggests that interdisciplinary review of individual cases, coupled with a systematic program to follow up child abuse case reports with telephone calls to the agencies designated to provide services to the children and families, is associated with lowering both the duration of hospitalization and the dollar cost of the medical treatment of child abuse, and with a reduction of the reinjury rate (101).

Of the evaluations of child abuse demonstration programs, two studies stand out. Cohn and her associates enlisted the cooperation of the grantees under a 1973 child abuse initiative (funded, interestingly, by the Nixon administration as part of an effort to convince Congress that the legislation to create a National Center on Child Abuse and Neglect was unnecessary) in documenting the process of the projects' development and their success in attaining their objectives. For the first and only time, data on individual cases served to assess the work of the projects. A salient finding particularly relevant to present-day approaches to child abuse was that lay intervention agents appeared to be as effective as child welfare professionals (102).

Daro recently reported the findings of the National Clinical Evaluation Study, which measured costs of services as well as certain indicators of outcome (103). Among the more important findings were the following: "The most cost-effective treatment plan in instances of child sexual abuse involving family members seems to be a combination of family and group counseling for the victim, the victim's siblings, the perpetrator and perpetrator's spouse. In cases of child neglect, the most efficient interventions will combine family counseling with parent education and basic care services such as babysitting, medical care, clothing and housing assistance" (p. 197). The author voices despair over the vast needs of victims of child abuse and their families and the paucity of resources committed to them and emphasizes the efficiencies implied in preventive approaches: "However, the prevailing evidence suggests that treatment efforts, at best, are successful with only half of their clients and that the poorest, most dysfunctional families are least likely to achieve successful outcomes. Given the high cost of treatment services and their limited promise for remediating the consequences of maltreatment, prevention efforts appear to be a more efficient alternative. Approximately $1.3 billion would purchase two years of weekly parenting education and supervised parent-child interactions for all adolescent mothers" (p. 198).

The opening sentence of Tolstoy's *Anna Karenina* frames the principal issue with which individual practitioners and architects of social policy must contend in contemplating what to do with victims of child abuse and family violence: "Happy families are all alike; every unhappy family is unhappy in its own way" (104). The many symptoms, and the multiplicity of causes, call for individualized responses once violence has occurred, both for the victim and for the family (104). These include

- medical and psychiatric diagnostic and therapeutic services
- social work diagnosis and treatment
- nursing service
- child care services and homemakers
- parenting services: parent aides, Parents Anonymous
- substitute care services
- legal initiatives: custody and criminal processes; other sanctions

When the choice of the appropriate interventions is made with thought and care, and when the services are indeed available, the outcomes for the children appear to be favorable (105). When they are not, damage both to child and family can ensue.

The paucity of resources for victims of child abuse and the prevailing low quality of child protection services in the United States have stimulated debate whether to restrict both the social welfare agencies and the courts in their decision prerogatives. With a view to protecting children and families from the possibly incompetent intrusions of state workers, restrictive standards for practice have been proposed, and the American Civil Liberties Union initiated two unsuccessful class action suits challenging the child welfare agencies' abilities to enter homes and to examine children without search warrants issued by courts (106–108). More restrictive and procedure-bound practices, however, might lead to further conflicts in the delivery of services to individual children and could culminate ultimately in a more intrusive pattern of practice as the courts—with attorneys arrayed in adversarial postures on behalf of agencies, parents, and children--would have to sort through the data on each case (109).

Prevention holds promise for reducing the impact and cost of child abuse, and with the appropriate evaluative effort should frame a national policy, in the view of many professional bodies, including an advisory committee to the National Center on Child Abuse and Neglect. Given the risks of reinjury and the consequences of child abuse, treatment can be understood also as a tertiary form of prevention, but no longer can we afford to neglect primary and secondary preventive initiatives. These can be organized in relation to theories of etiology. Several theories of prevention are outlined in the paragraphs that follow.

PREVENTION

From Psychoanalytic Theory

1. Acknowledge the importance of mental health to the functioning and well-being of children and families by formalizing a conception of health that includes emotional as well as biological health. This can be achieved through the training of physicians and others to recognize and attend to emotional as well as physiological issues in practice, and by providing third party reimbursement for serving as the patient's advisor, counselor, and health advocate (110).

From Learning Theory

2. Give parents access to information and understanding of child development, including nonviolent methods of socializing their children.

From Attachment Theory

3. Elevate the parent-child relationship to an appropriate position of respect and importance in clinical practice, by preventing prematurity through prenatal care, humanizing the delivery experience, bringing fathers into the delivery room and emphasizing their supportive role toward mothers and their participation in child care, and by encouragement of paternity leaves as well as maternity leaves from employment (111).

From Stress Theory

4. Provide hotlines to ensure quick telephone access for parents at times of distress with their children (112).

5. Make available to all children health and mental health services including well child care, diagnosis, and treatment.

6. Make available emergency homemaker and/or child care services to families in crisis.

7. Reduce social isolation by ensuring universal access to telephones and public transportation to facilitate social interactions.

8. Support existing community institutions (such as churches and women's organizations) that offer support, a sense of community, and feelings of self-worth to their members.

9. Empower women. Acknowledge the extent to which sexual dominance and subservience figures both in the abuse of women and children and in professional settings where male-dominated professions (medicine, surgery,

law) hold sway over professions composed mainly of women (social work, nursing, child care).

From Labeling Theory

10. Remove the stigma associated with getting help for family problems by detaching protective service programs from public welfare agencies. Abandon the heavily value-laden nomenclature of the "battered child syndrome," "child abuse," and "child neglect" in favor of a broader and more humane conception of childhood social illness. Increase the sensitivity, timeliness, and competency of medical and social work practice.

11. Expand public awareness of the prevalence of child abuse and domestic violence, and disassemble the conventional wisdom attaching child abuse to deviant and minority individuals and groups; emphasize that the potential for violence is in all of us; and put a priority on individual and social action to intervene when violence occurs.

These recommendations for the prevention of child physical abuse have been elaborated elsewhere in relation to the existing theory base on child abuse (113).

From Present Practice

The following steps to prevent child sexual abuse derive from the somewhat more limited present understanding of etiology, symptoms, and consequences:

1. Develop programs to educate children and professionals about sexual abuse. Children can be empowered to say no and to get help. Physicians, other medical workers, education, social service, and mental health professionals, if acquainted with the physical and behavioral signs of sexual victimization, can act early to prevent its serious consequences.

2. Diminish the culturally sanctioned sexual exploitation of children. The use of children as sexual lures to sell products by advertisers or to attract viewers to movies and other media should be discouraged by parents, professional organizations, and trade associations. Governmental initiatives must take cognizance of the constraints imposed by the first amendment of the Constitution, realizing that as with child pornography, when these efforts begin, they will almost certainly be challenged in the courts.

3. Screen professionals who work with children. Individuals who seek to exploit children through employment as day care and health workers, teachers, or clergy can be identified through careful interviewing and subsequent supervision on the job. Because most pedophiles do not have criminal records, fingerprints and criminal record screens will probably be unavailing. These methods may, indeed, discourage talented people from careers in child care. References can be obtained and checked, and reasons for choosing the work and special preferences for ages and genders of children can be explored. To date, no specific and sensitive methods for identifying adults who may sexually abuse children have been developed.

4. Protect child victims from traumatic court procedures. Only a third of the jurisdictions in the United States have promulgated guidelines for examining and interviewing sexually abused children. The education of prosecutors and judges might well include the development of lines of referral and consultation with skilled medical and mental health professionals (114).

REFERENCES

1. Kempe CH, Silverman FN, Steele BF, et al. The battered child syndrome. JAMA 1962; 181:17–24.
2. Gershenson CP. Child maltreatment and the federal role. In: Gil D, ed. Child abuse and violence. New York: AMS Press, 1979: 18–36.
3. Zigler E. Controlling child abuse in America: An effort doomed to failure. In: Bourne R. Newberger E, eds. Critical perspectives on child abuse. Lexington MA: Lexington Books, 1979: 171–213.
4. Newberger EH, Bourne R. The medicalization and legalization of child abuse. Am J Orthopsychiatry 1978; 48:593–607.
5. Kempe CH, Helfer RE, eds. Helping the battered child and his family. Philadelphia: Lippincott, 1972.
6. Cohen S, Sussman R. Reporting child abuse. Cambridge: Ballinger, 1977.
7. Price M. Child protection report. Washington, DC, March 13, 1975.
8. Carr A, Gelles RF. Reporting child maltreatment in Florida: The operation of public child protective service systems. Report submitted to the National Center on Child Abuse and Neglect, 1978.
9. Attorney General's Task Force on Family Violence. Final report. Washington, DC: US Dept. of Justice, 1984.
10. Strain JE (American Academy of Pediatrics). Decision to forego life-sustaining treatment for seriously ill newborns. Pediatrics 1983; 72:572–573.
11. Proposed regulations, Public Law 93-247, National Center on Child Abuse and Neglect. Federal Register. Washington, DC, April 24, 1985: 16105.
12. Bittner S, Newberger EH. Pediatric understanding of child abuse and neglect. Pediatrics 1981; 2:197–207.
13. Newberger EH, Reed RB, Daniel JH, et al. Pediatric social illness: Toward an etiologic classification. Pediatrics 1977; 60:178–185.
14. Newberger EH, Hampton RL, Marx TJ, White KN. Child abuse and pediatric social illness: An epidemiological analysis and ecological reformulation. Am J Orthopsychiatry 1986; 56:589–601.
15. White KN, Snyder J, Bourne R, Newberger EH. Treating child abuse and family violence in hospitals. Lexington, MA: Lexington Books, 1989.
16. Meadow R. Munchausen syndrome by proxy: The hinterland of child abuse. Lancet 1977; 2:343–344.
17. Meadow R. Munchausen syndrome by proxy. Arch Dis Child 1982; 57:92.
18. Rosen CL, Frost JD, Bricker T, et al. Two siblings with recurrent cardiorespiratory arrest. Munchausen syndrome by proxy or child abuse? Pediatrics 1983; 71:715–720.
19. Meadow R. Factitious epilepsy. Lancet 1984; 2:25–29.
20. Newberger CM, Newberger EH. When the pediatrician is a pedophile. In:

Burgess AW, Hartman CR eds. Sexual exploitation of patients by health professionals. New York: Praeger Press, 1986, 99–106.

21. Guandolo VL. Munchausen syndrome by proxy: An outpatient challenge. Pediatrics 1985; 75:526–536.

22. Finkelhor D. Child sexual abuse: New theory and research. New York: Free Press, 1984.

23. Burgess AW, ed. Child pornography and sex rings. Lexington, MA: Lexington Books, 1985.

24. McKibben L, DeVos E, Newberger EH. Victimization of mothers of abused children: A controlled study. Pediatrics 1989; 84:531–535.

25. Bassuk EL, Rosenberg L. Why does family homelessness occur? A case-control study. Am J Public Health 1988; 78:783–788.

26. Gelles RJ. Violence in the family: A review of research in the seventies. J Marriage and Family 1980; 42:873–878.

27. Gil DG. Violence against children: Physical child abuse in the United States. Cambridge: Harvard University Press, 1970.

28. Light RJ. Abused and neglected children in America. Harvard Ed Rev 1973; 43:556.

29. American Humane Association. Annual report of official child abuse and neglect reporting. Denver: American Humane Association, 1986.

30. Children's Defense Fund. A children's defense budget. Washington, DC: Children's Defense Fund, 1985.

31. Straus M, Gelles RJ, Steinmetz SK. Behind closed doors: Violence in the American family. New York: Doubleday, 1980.

32. Gelles RJ, Straus MA. Intimate violence. New York: Simon and Schuster, 1988.

33. US Dept of Health and Human Services. Study methodology: National study of the incidence and severity of child abuse and neglect. DHHS Pub No (OHDS) 81-30326. Washington. DC: US Govt. Printing Office, 1981.

34. Finklehor D, Hotaling GT. Sexual abuse in the national incidence study of child abuse and neglect: An appraisal. Child Abuse and Neglect 1984; 8:23–27.

35. Finkelhor D. Sexually victimized children. New York: Free Press, 1979.

36. Peters SD, Wyatt GE, Finkelhor D. Prevalence. In: Finkelhor D. A source book on child sexual abuse. Beverly Hills: Sage, 1986, 15–59.

37. Finkelhor D. Sex among siblings: A survey report on its prevalence, its variety, and its effects. Arch Sex Behavior 1980; 9:171.

38. Hampton RL, Newberger EH. Child abuse incidence and reporting by hospitals: Significance and severity, class, and race. Am J Public Health 1985; 75:56–60.

39. US Dept Health and Human Services. Study findings: Study of national incidence and prevalence of child abuse and neglect. Report of contract 105-85-1702. Washington, DC: DHHS, 1988.

40. Steele BF, Pollock C. A psychiatric study of parents who abuse infants and small children. In: Helfer RE, Kempe CH eds. The battered child. Chicago: University of Chicago Press, 1974, 80–133.

41. Helfer RE. Basic issues concerning prediction. In: Helfer RE, Kempe CH eds. Child abuse and neglect: The family and the community. Cambridge: Ballinger, 1976.

42. Garbarino J, Sherman D. Defining the community context for parent-child relations: The correlates of child maltreatment. Child Dev 1978; 49:604.

43. Garbarino J. The human ecology of child maltreatment: A conceptual model for research. J Marriage and Family 1977; 39:721–732.
44. Belsky J. The determinants of parenting: A process model. Child Dev 1984; 55:55–57.
45. Gelles RJ. Child abuse as psychopathology: A sociological critique and reformulation. Am J Orthopsychiatry 1973; 43:611–621.
46. Galdston R. Violence begins at home. Am J Child Psychiatry 1971; 10:336–350.
47. Parke RD, Collmer CW. Child abuse: An interdisciplinary analysis. In: Hetherington EM, ed. Review of child development research. Chicago: University of Chicago Press, 1975, 509–590.
48. Straus MA. Stress and physical child abuse. Child Abuse and Neglect 1980; 4:75.
49. Newberger CM, Cook S. Parental awareness and child abuse: A cognitive-developmental analysis of urban and rural samples. Am J Orthopsychiatry 1983; 53:512–524.
50. O'Toole R, Turbett, Nalepka C. Theories, professional knowledge, and diagnosis of child abuse. In: Finkelhor D, Gelles R, Hotaling GT, Straus MA, eds. The dark side of families: Current family violence research. Beverly Hills: Sage, 1983, 349–362.
51. Smith SM, Hanson R, Noble S. Parents of battered babies: A controlled study. Br Med J 1973; 4:388–391.
52. Spinetta J, Rigler D. The child abusing parent: A psychological review. Psychol Bull 1972; 77:296.
53. Starr RH. Controlled study of the ecology of child abuse and drug abuse. Child Abuse and Neglect 1978; 2:19–28.
54. Burgess RL, Draper P. The explanation of family violence: The role of biological, behavioral, and cultural selection. In: Ohlin L, Tonry M, eds. Family violence. Chicago: University of Chicago Press, 1989, 59–116.
55. Garbarino J, Gilliam G. Understanding abusive families. Lexington, MA: Lexington Books, 1980.
56. Zuravin S. Fertility patterns: Their relationship to child physical abuse and child neglect. J Marriage and Family 1988; 50:93–993.
57. Lynch MA. Ill-health and child abuse. Lancet 1975; 2:317–319.
58. Sherrod KB, O'Connor S, Vietze PM, et al. Child health and maltreatment. Child Dev 1984; 55:1174–1183.
59. Solomons G. Child abuse and developmental disabilities. Dev Med Child Neurol 1979; 21:101–106.
60. Klein M, Stern S. Low birth weight and the battered child syndrome. Am J Dis Child 1971; 122:15.
61. North Carolina Division of Social Services. Protective services for children, medical and medico-legal diagnostic studies and evaluations, processed. October 1, 1983.
62. Whitworth J, Lanier M, Skinner RG, Lund N. A multidisciplinary, hospital-based team for child abuse cases: A "hands-on" approach. Child Welfare 1981; 11:233–343.
63. Leventhal JM. Risk factors for child abuse: Methodologic standards in case-control studies. Pediatrics 1981; 63:684–690.
64. Egeland B, Vaughn B. Failure of "bond formation" as a cause of abuse, neglect, and maltreatment. Am J Orthopsychiatry 1981; 51:78–84.

65. Gelles RJ. Applying research on family violence to clinical practice. J Marriage and Family 1982; 44:9–20.
66. Dept of Social Services, Commonwealth of Massachusetts. Reference guide for child abuse and neglect investigations, 1985: 55.
67. Ellerstein NS. Child abuse: A medical reference. New York: Wiley, 1981.
68. Diamond LJ, Jaudes PK. Child abuse in a cerebral-palsied population. Dev Med Child Neurol 1983; 25:169.
69. Jason J, Gilliand JC, Tyler CW. Homicide as a cause of pediatric mortality in the United States. Pediatrics 1983; 72:191–193.
70. Jason J, Carpenter M, Tyler CW. Underreporting of infant homicide in the United States. Am J Public Health 1983; 73:195–197.
71. Rosenberg ML, Gelles RJ, Holinger PC, et al. Violence: Homicide, assault, and suicide. In: Ambler RW, Dull B, eds. Closing the gap. New York: Oxford University Press, 1987, 164–178.
72. White ST, Loda FA, Ingram DL, et al. Sexually transmitted diseases in sexually abused children. Pediatrics 1983; 72:16–21.
73. Canavan JW. Sexual child abuse. In: Ellerstein NS, ed. Child abuse: A medical reference. New York: Wiley, 1981, 233–251.
74. Kinnard EM. Emotional development in physically abused children. Am J Orthopsychiatry 1980; 50:686–696.
75. Lynch MA, Roberts R. Consequences of child abuse. New York: Academic Press, 1982.
76. Widom CS. Child abuse, neglect, and adult behavior: Research design and findings on criminality. Am J Orthopsychiatry 1989; 59:355–367.
77. Elmer E. A followup study of traumatized children. Pediatrics 1977; 59:273.
78. McCord J. A thirty-year followup of treatment effects. Am Psychol 1978; 33:284.
79. McCord W, McCord J. Origins of crime: A new evaluation of the Cambridge-Somerville Youth Study. New York: Columbia University Press, 1959.
80. Vosburgh WW, Alexander LB. Long-term followup as program evaluation: Lessons from McCord's 30 year followup of the Cambridge-Somerville Youth Study. Am J Orthopsychiatry 1980; 50:109–124.
81. McCord J. A forty-year perspective on effects of child abuse and neglect. Child Abuse and Neglect 1983; 7:265–270.
82. Wyatt GE, Powell GJ. Lasting effects of child sexual abuse. Newbury Park, CA: Sage, 1988.
83. Sedney M, Brooks B. Factors associated with a history of childhood sexual experience in a nonclinical population. J Am Acad Child Psychiatry 1984; 23:215.
84. Summit R, Kryso J. Sexual abuse of children: A clinical spectrum. Am J Orthopsychiatry 1978; 48:237–251.
85. Div of Child Psychiatry, Tufts New England Medical Center. Sexually exploited children: Service and research project. Final report to the Office of Juvenile Justice and Delinquency Prevention. Washington, DC: US Dept. of Justice, 1984.
86. Straus M. Behavioral consequences of sexual victimization (unpublished master's thesis). University of Maryland, 1980.
87. Browne A, Finkelhor D. The impact of child sexual abuse: A review of the research. Psych Bull 1986; 99:66–77.
88. Nemiah JC. Dissociative disorders. In: Kaplan HI, Sadock BJ, eds. Compre-

hensive textbook of psychiatry, 4th ed. Baltimore: Williams and Wilkins, 1984, 942–957.

89. Putnam FW, ed. Multiple personality. Psychiatric Ann 1984; 14:1.

90. Finkelhor D. The sexual abuse of boys. Victimology 1981; 6:76.

91. Steele B, Alexander H. Long-term effects of sexual abuse in childhood. In: Mrazek PB, Kempe CH, eds. Sexually abused children and their families. Oxford: Pergamon Press, 1981.

92. Groth A, Birnbaum J. Men who rape: A psychology of the offender. New York: Plenum Press, 1979.

93. Meiselman K. Incest: A psychological study of the causes and effects with treatment recommendations. San Francisco: Jossey-Bass, 1978.

94. Newberger CM, DeVos E. Abuse and victimization: A life-span developmental perspective. Am J Orthopsychiatry 1988; 58:505–511.

95. Sherman LW, Berk RA. The Minneapolis domestic violence equipment. Washington, DC: Police Foundation Reports, April 1984.

96. Weiss EH, Berg RF. Child victim of sexual assault: Impact of court procedures. Am J Child Psychiatry 1982; 21:513–518.

97. Massachusetts Committee for Children and Youth. Newsletter, Spring 1985.

98. Runyan DK, Gould CL, Trost DC, et al. Determinants of foster care placement for the maltreated child. Am J Public Health 1981; 71:706–711.

99. Fanshel D. Decision-making under uncertainty: Foster care for abused and neglected children? Am J Public Health 1981; 71:685–686.

100. Davoren E. The profession of social work and the protection of children. In: Newberger E, ed. Child abuse. Boston: Little, Brown, 1982, 157–173.

101. Newberger EH, Hagenbuch JJ, Ebeling NB, et al. Reducing the literal and human cost of child abuse: Impact of a new hospital management system. Pediatrics 1973; 51:840–848.

102. Cohn AH. Evaluation of Child Abuse and Neglect Demonstration Projects, 2 vol. Washington, DC: DHHS, National Center for Health Services Research, 1978.

103. Daro D. Confronting child abuse: Research for effective program design. New York: Free Press, 1988.

104. Newberger EH, Bourne R. Preface. In: Newberger E, Bourne R, eds. Unhappy families: Clinical and research perspectives on family violence. Littleton, MA: PSG, 1985.

105. Cohn AH. Effective treatment of child abuse and neglect. Soc Work 1979; 24:513–519.

106. American Civil Liberties Union of Illinois. EZ versus Kohler, Federal District Court, 1983.

107. American Civil Liberties Union of Massachusetts. Buckman et al. versus Matava, Massachusetts Superior Court, 1985.

108. Juvenile Justice Standards Project. Standards relating to abuse and neglect. Cambridge: Ballinger, 1977.

109. Bourne R, Newberger EH. Family autonomy or coercive intervention? Ambiguity and conflict in the proposed standards for child abuse and neglect. Boston Univ Law Rev 1977; 57:670–706.

110. Almy TP. The role of the primary physician in the health care industry. New Engl J Med 1981; 304:225–228.

111. Garbarino J. Changing hospital childbirth practices: A developmental perspective on prevention of child maltreatment. Am J Orthopsychiatry 1979; 49:588–597.

112. National Center on Child Abuse and Neglect. Child abuse helplines: A special report from the National Center on Child Abuse and Neglect. Washington, DC: DHHS, 1979.
113. Newberger CM, Newberger EH. Prevention of child abuse: Theory, myth, practice. J Prev Psychiatry 1982; 1:443–451.
114. Bulkley J, ed. Innovations in the prosecution of child sexual abuse cases. Washington, DC: National Legal Resource Center for Child Advocacy and Protection, American Bar Association, 1981.

4

Child Sexual Abuse

DAVID FINKELHOR

Child sexual abuse is sexual contact with a child that occurs as a result of force or in a relationship where it is exploitative because of an age difference or caretaking responsibility. There were an estimated 155,900 cases of child sexual abuse identified by professionals in 1986, a 221 percent increase over 1980. However, research on this subject is difficult, scarce, and extremely variable in quality.

The best sense of the true scope of the problem comes from community surveys that elicited reports from adults of past experiences. These surveys indicate that from 6 percent to 62 percent of women and 2 percent to 15 percent of men have experienced child sexual abuse, that a third to two-fifths of these experiences occur with other family members, and one out of 12 with a father or stepfather. The peak ages of vulnerability appear to be between 9 and 12, but as many as a quarter of these incidents occur before the child is eight years of age.

Studies have failed to find higher risks for any racial or socioeconomic group. However, children whose parents are absent, unavailable, or in conflict, and children who have step-parents or poor relationships with their parents appear to be at higher risk.

Abusers are predominantly males. Studies of incarcerated offenders have confirmed: (1) unusual needs for domination, (2) unusual sexual arousal patterns, (3) histories of victimization, (4) conflicts in adult heterosexual relationships, and (5) drinking problems.

Recent studies reveal that women who were sexually abused as children have rates of mental health impairment almost twice as high as nonabused women. The long-term effects most clearly associated with child sexual abuse are depression, drug and alcohol abuse, sexual problems, and repeated victimization.

There has been broad public and professional mobilization around the problem since the early 1980s concentrating on public and professional education to increase reporting, preventive education for children in schools, and specialized treatment programs for victims and families. Other interventions include treatment programs for offenders and reforms in criminal justice procedures for handling sexual abuse. There have been almost no evaluations of these programs.

STATEMENT OF THE PROBLEM

The term *child sexual abuse* as it is commonly used in North America means sexual activity (single acts or extended contacts) involving a child that occurs (1) in a relationship where it is deemed exploitative by virtue of an age difference or caretaking relationship that exists with a child, and/or (2) as a result of force or threat. In both professional and popular terms, there is almost universal agreement that sexual contact between a child and his or her father, stepfather, mother, stepmother, another older relative, teacher, or babysitter constitutes sexual abuse. Sexual contact by any adult or older person, whether known or unknown, is also considered sexual abuse. And rape and forced sexual contact at the hands of anyone, even a peer, is generally included.

Not everyone uses this definition of sexual abuse, however, and within this definition there is not universal agreement about the exact boundaries of various terms. The National Center on Child Abuse and Neglect (NCCAN) and related child welfare agencies within individual states tend to restrict their "official definition" of child sexual abuse to activity at the hands of *caretakers* (1). This restriction, designed in part to separate state child welfare functions from criminal justice functions, excludes molestations by strangers.

Other writers and researchers limit child sexual abuse to contacts with adults, excluding forced sex that may take place at the hands of other children (2). Although there is some evidence that abuse by other children is not as traumatic as abuse by adults, many children suffer serious rapes and ongoing sexual abuse from older siblings, neighbors, and schoolmates (3). There is an increasing consensus among professionals to include such experiences in definitions of child sexual abuse for both research and treatment.

There are other specific definitional disagreements. (1) What is a "child"? Some definitions include persons up to the age of 18, although 16 is the more common demarcation in law and in practice (4). (2) What is an exploitive "age difference"? State laws codify this in a variety of ways in their statutory rape statutes (4). "Statutory" rape, according to the Federal Bureau of Investigation (FBI) definition, is rape without force. The most sophisticated laws use a sliding differential depending on the age of the younger partner. (3) What "sexual activities" are included? Although intercourse and genital touching are universally included, some definitions of sexual abuse involve the acts of an exposer and others require actual physical contact. Most definitions of child sexual abuse now include the use of children in prostitution and pornography.

Unfortunately, state statutes have not been of much assistance in clearly defining sexual abuse. In general they are extremely varied, complicated, and currently in flux (4). The pertinent criminal laws involve a mixture of offenses including rape, statutory rape, sodomy, indecent liberties, and incest with terminology like "carnal knowledge" and "lewd and lascivious acts." All states but one now include sexual abuse in their laws requiring the reporting of child abuse and neglect, but sexual abuse is rarely defined here either. Under recommendation from the American Bar Association, many states are finally moving to adopt specific definitions of child sexual abuse in their criminal codes (5).

DATA SOURCES

In the United States, police, child protective services, and medical facilities are the main agencies that document reports of sexual abuse. Numerous studies have been done on samples from all these sources (6-10). The largest and most comprehensive ongoing data collection was conducted from 1976 through 1987 by the American Humane Association. This data set collates on a nationwide basis state reports of child abuse and neglect including sexual abuse (11). In addition, the National Center on Child Abuse and Neglect commissioned two National Incidence Studies (NIS 1 and NIS 2) in 1981 and 1986, which gathered reports of sexual abuse and other kinds of child abuse and neglect from selected counties systematically chosen to represent the country (1,12). Other important data on sexual abuse come from mental health facilities where victims of sexual abuse seek treatment (13-16). Many studies, mostly in prison settings, have been conducted of sexual abusers (17,18). Studies of adults in the "normal" population, either students or the community at large, have focused on uncovering individuals with histories of sexual abuse (19-25).

Available Data Sources and Their Limitations

All the data sources on child sexual abuse have serious problems. Fear of prosecution on the part of offenders, together with embarrassment and shame on the part of victims and their families, all conspire to create serious obstacles to valid and reliable data. Some of the advantages and disadvantages of specific data sources are as follows:

1. The national data collected by the American Humane Association from state child protective agencies constitutes a very large sample collected over a number of years using uniform definitions and protocols (11). However, there are relatively few variables relating to each case, and more seriously, these "reported" cases constitute only a fraction of all occurrences

of child sexual abuse (26). The exact fraction these reported cases constitute is difficult to estimate, but it is certainly less than one-third (21).

2. Aggregate data from the criminal justice system have not been readily usable. In the past, the Uniform Crime Reports collected by the Federal Bureau of Investigation have not included the age of victim as a variable, making it impossible to distinguish child sexual abuse from other sexual assaults. Moreover, the variability of laws that define sexual abuse for criminal justice purposes in different states has made it very difficult to compare criminal justice system data across states or even within one state. Finally, the cases coming to the attention of the criminal justice system as well as to the medical system constitute an even smaller proportion of actual cases than those reported to the child welfare reporting agencies.

3. The two National Incidence Studies on Child Abuse and Neglect (1,12) generated sexual abuse data that had some of the same limitations as the data already available from the American Humane Association (26). Each NIS recorded only cases known to professionals, and it collected limited information on each case.

4. Descriptive studies of offenders have suggested hypotheses about the motivations for sexual abuse, but many of these studies are seriously limited by the inclusion of only incarcerated offenders. Only a very small and unrepresentative fraction of offenders end up in prison: those who are most repetitive in their offending, those who have prior criminal records, those who are poor and unable to afford effective defense counsel, and those who commit violent offenses against non-family members (17).

5. Community surveys constitute the most representative data collection efforts (14,23–25), gathering information on the estimated 75–90 percent of cases that are never reported to any agency. But such surveys are expensive, and there are unanswered questions about the reliability and validity of the data they gather. In addition, when adults are questioned about abuses they suffered as children, there is probably some distortion due to memory loss. There is also undoubtedly withholding of information in these surveys, and it is hard to know how much. Most problematic is the fact that, because they are surveys of adults, the data can not necessarily be generalized to the current generation of children, for whom rates and circumstances of victimization may be very different. Dependent young children have not been surveyed because of the risk that an abusing parent, discovering that a child had told, might in anger cause the child great harm.

Developing Better Data Sources

Perhaps the most important need in this field is for an ongoing national data collection system with uniform standards and mandated participation. There are such national systems for reports of diseases and also for reports of crimes, but none as yet for child welfare data.

In addition, large community surveys of young adults and older adolescents would be one of the most useful ways to better estimate the amount and nature of the great amount of child sexual abuse that still goes unreported. These respondents would be close enough to their experiences to give more accurate data that would be historically relevant. At the same time, they would be emancipated enough to give information about abuse experiences without danger of retaliation from their abusers. The possibility of surveying dependent young children should not be ruled out entirely. This might be feasible if research were combined with extremely sensitive efforts to screen for and then intervene in the cases of ongoing abuse that were discovered in the study. Another important research need is for longitudinal studies that follow a cohort of children to determine which ones become the victims of sexual abuse and how this affects their development. Finally, there is a strong need for case-control studies of offenders and nonoffenders to find out more about the sources of abusive behavior among a representative sample of abusers (incarcerated and nonincarcerated).

RISK FACTORS AND CAUSES

Prevalence and Characteristics

The best sense of the scope of child sexual abuse comes from community surveys of normal adults. These studies have found that at least 5 percent of adults report some sexual abuse in their childhood, but the variation among the studies is great and the reported incidence ranges from 6 percent to 62 percent for women and from 2 percent to 15 percent for men. For example, in one of the largest and most meticulous studies, Russell surveyed a random sample of 933 women in San Francisco and found 38 percent had been sexually abused before the age of 18; 16 percent had been abused by a family member (23). In the only national survey of child sexual abuse to date, conducted by the Los Angeles Times Poll among 2,626 Americans, 27 percent of the women and 16 percent of the men reported having been abused (25). By contrast, in a phone sample of 603 Nashville area residents, a survey research firm elicited histories of sexual abuse from only 11 percent of the women (27). A number of other studies of normal populations have been done with varying degrees of sophistication (19–22).

This variation in reported rates reflects a variety of factors: (1) different studies use different definitions of sexual abuse, although those with more encompassing definitions do not necessarily produce higher estimates, (2) there are probably real differences in the extent of victimization in different geographic areas and different population subgroups, (3) the way in which investigators select subjects and ask questions about an extremely sensitive subject like sexual abuse undoubtedly has a large influence on estimates.

So far it would appear that studies using extended, in-person interviews have achieved higher (and presumably more valid) estimates than those using telephone interviews or self-administered questionnaires (28). Moreover, studies that have used a large number of specific screening questions within which an experience of sexual abuse might be reported (for example, "Were you ever forced to have intercourse?" or "Did you ever have unwanted sexual contact with a person in authority?") produce more positive reports than those using single broad and unspecific screening questions ("Were you ever sexually abused as a child?") (28). Considering additional factors, such as the likelihood of memory loss and some degree of intentional concealment, the true national prevalence for women who were sexually abused by age 16 (including abuse by peers but excluding experiences with exposers) probably runs in the range of 25 percent to 40 percent (28).

Community studies are also the best sources of information about the prevalence and characteristics of different types of sexual abuse (19,21,23–25,27). These studies suggest that abuse by fathers and stepfathers, even though it dominates reports from the child welfare system, actually constitutes no more than 7–8 percent of all abuse cases. Abuse by other family members (most frequently uncles and older brothers) constitutes an additional 16–42 percent. Other nonrelatives known to the child (including neighbors, family friends, child care workers, and other authorities) make up 32 percent to 60 percent of offenders. Abuse by strangers (the traditional stereotype of the child molester), making up the remainder, is in almost all studies substantially less common than abuse either by family members or by persons known to the child.

The largest category of abuse in most studies involves groping or fondling of children's bodies on top of or underneath the clothing. Only 16–29 percent of the abuse involves intercourse or attempted intercourse. Another 3–11 percent of the activities involve attempted or completed oral or anal intercourse, and 13–33 percent, manual touching of the genitals.

Community studies show the frequency of child sexual abuse seems to peak when victims are between ages 9 and 12, and then declines somewhat during later adolescent years. (This distribution changes somewhat, however, depending on how much of adolescent date and acquaintance rape is included as sexual abuse.) Most studies show that a quarter of the incidents occur among victims under eight years of age, and some clinicians insist that this percentage would be even greater if it were not for the occlusion of memories from these early years (29). Approximately 42–75 percent of experiences reported in the surveys are single events that did not reoccur. Repeated abusive experiences occur at older ages and are associated with abuse within the family.

In addition to community surveys, compilations of "officially reported" cases have been used to generate incidence estimates and describe other characteristics of child sexual abuse. For example, the National Incidence Study 2 (12) projected that 155,900 new cases of sexual abuse became known to professionals in the United States in 1986. Incidence estimates based on reported cases such as these appear to overrepresent (1) abuse involving fathers and stepfathers, (2) abuse involving intercourse and other more intrusive acts, and (3) abuse perpetrated over an extended period. The ages of the victimized children also tend to be higher, since these reported cases record the age at the time of the disclosure rather than the age at onset.

Compared to the community studies, there also seems to be an underreporting of the sexual abuse of boys (21).

The number of reported cases of child sexual abuse in the United States has been growing dramatically since 1976 (30) and showed a 221 percent increase between 1980 and 1986 (31). However, this may not represent a true increase in incidence in recent years, but may have resulted primarily from the intensification of case detection efforts through media exposure and professional education. It should be noted that several of the community studies do not tend to show higher rates of sexual abuse among youngest cohorts (23–25).

Sociodemographic Distribution

Community surveys have provided information about the distribution of sexual abuse within various sociodemographic subgroups in the communities studied (21–25,27,32). These studies consistently fail to find differences in rates among different social classes or races.

However, several other factors have emerged from the community studies as being consistently associated with a higher risk for abuse: (1) when the child lives without one of the biological parents, (2) when the mother is unavailable to the child either as a result of employment outside the home or because of disability or illness, (3) when the child reports that the parents' marriage is unhappy or full of conflict, (4) when the child reports having a poor relationship with the parents or being subject to extremely punitive discipline or child abuse, (5) when the child reports having a stepfather (32). Although few studies have examined why these factors increase risk, poor supervision, emotional turmoil, neglect, and rejection may make a child vulnerable to the ploys of child molesters. In other words, as a result of conflicts and emotional deficits, the children are easier to manipulate with offers of affection, attention, and rewards in exchange for sex and secrecy. Unable to count on help and support from parents, these children may also find it harder for them to stop the abuse once it begins.

Research on Offenders

One clearly established fact about offenders is that they are predominantly males. This finding has been confirmed in nonclinical studies and in large-scale surveys of sexual histories undertaken to study questions other than child sexual abuse. A comprehensive review reported that women are perpetrators in no more than 5 percent of the abuse cases involving girls and 20 percent of the cases involving boys and that these proportions are not the result of reporting or labeling biases (33). This disproportionate perpetration by men clearly distinguishes sexual abuse from other forms of child abuse and neglect.

A wide variety of theories has been proposed to account for abusers, mostly on the basis of clinical experience with incarcerated offenders (18,34,35).

These theories can be organized into four categories or dynamics, according to whether they argue that abusers abuse (1) because they get powerful, developmentally induced emotional gratification from the acts, (2) because they have deviant physiological sexual arousal patterns, (3) because they are blocked in their capacity to meet their sexual needs in more conventional ways, or (4) because they have problems in their capacity for behavioral inhibition. Although often presented as competing theories, several of these dynamics may be present simultaneously, and different dynamics may be present in different types of molesting behavior.

There is some reasonable empirical support for some of these theories: (1) most groups of offenders who have been tested using physiological monitors (36–39) do show unusual levels of deviant sexual arousal to children, (2) many offenders have their own histories of having been victims of sexual abuse, although it is far from universal, tending to average between 25 percent and 33 percent (40–44), (3) many offenders do have conflicts over adult heterosexual relationships or are experiencing disruption in normal adult heterosexual partnerships at the time of offense (43,45,46), (4) alcohol is related to the commission of 19–70 percent of the offenses in a large number of studies, although no causative role for alcohol has been established (47,48).

A review (49) of studies of incestuous fathers, a group of particular interest to the child welfare system, finds evidence for the contention that such men (1) have difficulties in empathy, nurturance, and caretaking, and (2) are socially isolated and lacking in social skills. They are more frequently victims of physical abuse than sexual abuse and have poor relationships with their own fathers. They tend to be weakly identified with traditional masculine roles.

A particularly noteworthy study of incestuous abuse found that fathers who committed incest had participated less actively in early care of their victim children than had a comparison group of normal fathers, suggesting that early interaction with a young and dependent child may create some inhibitions against seeing this child as a sex object later on (50). Another recent study suggests that sexual abusers have histories of sexual deviance and deviant fantasies that generally go back to adolescence (51). This study also found a much greater extent and variety of deviant sexual acts among child molesters than had been previously reported. In summary, there are some promising leads, but research on sexual child abusers is in an extremely primitive state.

OUTCOMES

Impact of Sexual Abuse

Clinicians in the United States and Canada have noted many symptoms in children who have been sexually abused. These include fear, compulsivity, hyperactivity, phobias, withdrawal, guilt, depression, mood swings, suicidal ideation, fatigue, loss of appetite, somatic complaints, changes in sleeping and eating patterns, hostility, mistrust, sexual acting out, dissociative disorders, compulsive masturbation, and school problems (52–54). However, there have been very few systematic evaluations of large samples of sexually abused children to assess the prevalence and seriousness of these various symptoms. One exception was the Tufts Family Crisis Program study, which evaluated 113 sexually abused children within a year after disclosure using standardized psychological measures (16). Seventy percent of 4- to 6-year-olds met criteria for clinically significant pathology on the Louisville Behavior Checklist, as did 40 percent of the 7- to 13-year-olds. The most commonly observed symptomatic behaviors among the school-age abused children were aggression (50%), antisocial behavior (45%), fear (45%), immaturity (40%), neurotic behavior (38%), and sexual behavior (36%). Fearfulness, anger, and hostility are the most common observations in other such studies. In another systematic study of 369 abused children, children from poorly functioning families and children who did not have a supportive relationship with some adult showed a larger number of symptoms (55). Children involved in lengthy unresolved criminal cases also appear to stay symptomatic for longer periods (56).

In contrast to these initial effects, the long-term impact of sexual abuse has been the subject of more sophisticated studies. Various surveys of sexually abused women in the general population have all found significant, identifiable mental health impairment in victims compared to nonvictims in the same samples (3,19,21,23,57–59). One of the best was a survey of 344 women in Calgary using standardized epidemiological measures (19). This study found sexually abused women to have about twice the risk for depression, psychoneurosis, somatic anxiety, psychiatric hospitalization, and suicidal gestures. Moreover, sexual abuse was demonstrated to be a major risk for such outcomes even when controlling for other negative developmental and family background factors. However, severe levels of psychopathology were apparent in less than 25 percent of the sexual abuse victims. Another epidemiological survey (60) found two to three times the rate of psychiatric morbidity among adults molested as children, men as well as women.

Other studies have yielded similar findings. In a random sample of 250 Los Angeles women, Peters found that a history of sexual abuse was associated with an increased risk for depression, as well as for drug and alcohol abuse, even when background factors were controlled (58). Two other outcomes uncovered by studies in the general population are sexual problems—including frigidity, vaginismus or pain upon intercourse, flashbacks, and other emotional problems related to sex—and a much higher risk of subsequent sexual victimization (14,23,57,61,62).

Studies that have compared sexual abuse victims to other help-seekers in various clinical populations have also found sexual abuse victims to be more impaired on a number of dimensions (12–15,63): victims experienced more isolation, lower self-esteem, fear of men, anxiety attacks, sleeping difficulties, nightmares, alcohol and drug abuse, and were more prone to suicide and self-mutilation. Additional research suggests connections between sexual abuse and prostitution (64,65), multiple personality disorder, and eating disorders (66). In short, these studies contribute to very rapidly mounting evidence of negative mental health outcomes for victims of child sexual abuse. None of the studies by themselves is definitive on this point, but the weight of the growing number of studies is impressive.

Given such evidence of serious effects on some individuals, researchers have now begun to look at whether certain aspects of the experience or the context of the experience may explain the degree of trauma. However, this research is still very tentative (52). The weight of current evidence is that victims show more long-term symptoms when the abuse involves fathers and stepfathers (3,19,67), sexual intercourse (19,23), and force (3,19,57,67). In contrast, studies have not been able to demonstrate consistently that abuse at any particular age is more traumatic. One study of initial effects in children (16) shows that the factors predictive of greater disturbance are (1) violence and physical injury in the abusive episode, (2) a mother's hostile attitude toward the child upon revelation of the abuse, and (3) removal of the child from his or her home subsequent to the abuse. Unfortunately, research to date does not yet provide a clear basis for designating those types of abuse that should receive priority for professional attention.

INTERVENTIONS

Professional efforts to respond to the problem of sexual abuse can be grouped into the categories discussed in the paragraphs that follow:

Public Awareness
There have been broad campaigns in public and professional education designed to increase the detection and disclosure of sexual abuse. Books, brochures, and training programs for professionals, together with media coverage aimed at the public, have resulted in increased awareness of the problem. One effect of this awareness has been a rapid growth in the number of cases being reported to authorities.

However, this growth has raised many questions about policy. Child welfare agencies have been flooded with more cases than they can handle, and no criteria have been firmly established for how to prioritize reported cases for investigation. Moreover, many allegations of sexual abuse are extremely difficult to confirm, and there have been no studies concerning the reliability of various means of substantiating reports. One specific current controversy revolves around children's credibility. There is a consensus among professionals that children's allegations of abuse are mostly truthful, and that most subsequent recantations result from the pressure, fear, and stress that the children experience (68). However, under certain unusual conditions children may make distorted allegations, and there is not yet consensus about how to identify when these distortions occur. Finally, although most public and professional information on sexual abuse urges disclosure, it is also true that disclosure is extremely stressful on victims and families. Studies are badly needed to better understand the effects of disclosure and to evaluate procedures for minimizing these effects.

Preventive Education

A variety of educational programs have appeared, particularly within school systems, aimed at making children better able to protect themselves against victimization (69). Preventive education has been incorporated into hundreds of study books, comic books, coloring books, films, theatrical performances, and guides for teachers and parents. The intent of this material is to (1) explain what sexual abuse is, (2) inform children that they have a right and an obligation to refuse such activity, and (3) encourage them to tell someone about it.

These programs are extremely popular because they provide professionals and parents with special techniques for coping with the increasing public anxiety about the risk of sexual abuse. However, there is little research on their effectiveness in preventing abuse. Evaluations of several programs have demonstrated that children learn the concepts and do report previous incidents (70–72), but research has not yet established that such programs actually reduce the amount of later victimization.

Treatment Programs for Victims and Their Families

Specialized programs providing family, individual, and group treatment have been established in many communities by a wide range of agencies, including family service, mental health, and protective service agencies, hospitals, and probation and parole departments (73). The goals of these programs are generally to give support to victims and families in the aftermath of the disclosure and reduce the potential for long-term trauma. These programs use a mixture of individual, family, and group counseling techniques (74).

Very little research has been carried out to evaluate the effectiveness of specific types of interventions with victims and families. One particularly important policy question is whether to reunite children after treatment with parents who sexually abused them. Some argue that this reunification is ultimately healing for the children; others argue that it only increases the risk for further sexual and psychological abuse.

Treatment Programs for Offenders

There are a few dozen specialized, experimental child molester treatment programs around the country. Although programs have been established both within and outside of criminal justice settings, it has generally been found that the threat or reality of criminal sanctions must be utilized to assure the participation of offenders and to keep them away from victims. These programs employ a diversity of techniques including individual and group psychotherapy, behavior modification, social skills training, and some drug treatment (75).

Although there are many research reports of successful treatment of child molesters (51,76)—in particular, using behavior modification—a great deal of skepticism is warranted about the state of the art. Few sufficiently long-term follow-up studies have been done (77,78), especially given the evidence that recidivism often occurs many years subsequent to release (79). Moreover, it is generally acknowledged that some offenders are not amenable to treatment, and no reliable techniques exist for identifying these offenders.

Reforms of the Criminal Justice System

A variety of reforms have been proposed to reduce additional trauma to victims and to ensure more effective sanctions against offenders (80). Adoption of the proposals, however, has been slow and sporadic. These changes have included the use of videotaped testimony by children, victim advocates to assist victims and their families during the court process, diversion programs to encourage guilty pleas by offenders, restraining orders to remove offenders from the household thus avoiding removal of the child, expediting prosecution in sexual abuse cases, and redrafting of criminal statutes and their associated penalties. There is also an increasingly strong belief that for the sake of the victim it is important that criminal justice authorities work cooperatively with child protective, mental health, and medical personnel. Research is needed on how these criminal justice reforms actually affect the conviction, sentencing, and recidivism of offenders. Finally, public enthusiasm may be great for making the criminal justice process less traumatic to children in sex abuse cases, but there is no research to suggest how often children are traumatized by this process or which aspects of the process create trauma.

ANNOTATED BIBLIOGRAPHY

Faller K. Child sexual abuse: an interdisciplinary manual for diagnosis, case management, and treatment. New York: Columbia University Press, 1988.
This is an up-to-date manual on intervention and treatment.
Finkelhor D. Child sexual abuse: new theory and research. New York: Free Press, 1984.
This presents a comprehensive theory about the problem.
Finkelhor D et al, ed. Sourcebook on child sexual abuse. Beverly Hills, CA: Sage, 1986.
This book summarizes of research findings on prevalence, risk factors, the characteristics of offenders, and the impact on victims.
Russell D. The secret trauma: incest in the lives of girls and women. New York: Basic Books, 1986.
The best single study based on adult retrospective information with a great deal of powerful personal case information.

REFERENCES

1. National Center on Child Abuse and Neglect. National study of incidence and severity of child abuse and neglect. Washington, DC: National Center on Child Abuse and Neglect (NCCAN), 1981.
2. MacFarlane K, Jones B, Jenstrom L. Sexual abuse of children: Selected readings. Pub. no. 78-30161. Washington, DC: US Dept. of Health and Human Services, 1980.
3. Finkelhor D. Sexually victimized children. New York: Free Press, 1979.
4. Kocen L, Bulkley J. Analysis of criminal child sex offense statutes. In: Bulkley J, ed. Child sexual abuse and the law. Washington DC: American Bar Association, 1981: 1–51.
5. Bulkley J. Recommendations for improving legal intervention in intrafamily child sexual abuse cases. Washington DC: American Bar Association, 1981: 1–51.
6. Burgess AW, Groth AN, Holmstrom LL, Sgroi SM. Sexual assault of children and adolescents. Lexington, MA: Lexington Books, 1978.
7. DeFrancis V. Protecting the child victim of sex crimes committed by adults. Denver: American Humane Association, 1969.
8. Griffith S, Anderson S, Bach C, Paperny D. Intrafamily sexual abuse of male children: An underreported problem. Paper presented at the Third International Congress of Child Abuse and Neglect, Amsterdam, 1981.
9. Jaffe AC, Dynneson L, Ten Bensel R. Sexual abuse: An epidemiological study. Am J Dis Child 1975; 129:689–692.
10. Queen's Bench Foundation. Sexual abuse of children. San Francisco: Queen's Bench Foundation, 1976.
11. American Association for Protecting Children, Inc. National study on child neglect and abuse reporting. Denver: American Humane Association, 1984.
12. National Center on Child Abuse and Neglect. Study findings: Study of the national incidence and prevalence of child abuse and neglect. Washington, DC: US Dept. of Health and Human Services, 1988.
13. Briere J. The effect of childhood sexual abuse on later psychological functioning: Defining a "post-sexual-abuse syndrome." Paper presented at the Third National Conference on Sexual Victimization of Children, Washington, DC, April 1984.
14. Herman JL. Father-daughter incest. Cambridge: Harvard University Press, 1981.
15. Meiselman K. Incest: A psychological study of causes and effects with treatment recommendations. San Francisco: Jossey-Bass, 1978.
16. Tufts New England Medical Center, Division of Child Psychiatry. Sexually exploited children: Service and research project. Final report for the Office of Juvenile Justice and Delinquency Prevention, US Dept. of Justice, Boston, 1984.
17. Araji S, Finkelhor D. Explanations of pedophilia: Review of empirical evidence. Bulletin of the American Academy of Psychiatry and the Law 1985; 13:17–38.
18. Finkelhor D, Araji S. Explanations of pedophilia: A four factor model. J Sex Research 1986; 22(2):145–161.
19. Bagley C, Ramsay R. Disrupted childhood and vulnerability to sexual assault: Long-term sequels with implications for consulting. Social Work and Human Sexuality 1985; 4:33–48.

20. Committee on Sexual Offenses Against Children and Youth. Sexual offenses against children: Vol. 1. Ottawa: Canadian Government Publishing Centre, 1984.

21. Finkelhor D. Child sexual abuse: New theory and research. New York: Free Press, 1984.

22. Kercher G, McShane M. The prevalence of child sexual abuse victimization in an adult sample of Texas residents. Child Abuse Neglect 1984; 8(4):495–502.

23. Russell DEH. The secret trauma: Incest in the lives of girls and women. New York: Basic Books, 1986.

24. Wyatt G. The sexual abuse of Afro-American and White American women in childhood. Child Abuse Neglect 1985; 9:507–519.

25. Finkelhor D, Hotaling G, Lewis I, Smith C. Sexual abuse in a national survey of adult men and women: Prevalence, characteristics and risk factors. Child Abuse Neglect 1990; 14:19–28.

26. Finkelhor D, Hotaling G. Sexual abuse in the national incidence study of child abuse and neglect. Child Abuse Neglect 1984; 8:22–32.

27. Keckley Market Research. Sexual abuse in Nashville: A report on incidence and long-term effects. Nashville: Keckley Market Research, 1983.

28. Peters S, Wyatt G, Finkelhor D. The prevalence of child sexual abuse. In: Finkelhor D, et al, ed. A sourcebook on child sexual abuse. Beverly Hills, CA: Sage, 1986: 15–59.

29. Herman J. Personal communication, 1985.

30. Russell AB, Mohr-Trainor C. Trends in child abuse and neglect: A national perspective. Denver: American Humane Association, 1984.

31. National Committee for the Prevention of Child Abuse. The size of the child abuse problem. Working paper 008. Chicago: NCPCA, 1985.

32. Finkelhor D, Baron L. High risk children. In: Finkelhor D et al, ed. A sourcebook on child sexual abuse. Beverly Hills, CA: Sage, 1986: 60–88.

33. Finkelhor D, Russell DE. Women as perpetrators: Review of the evidence. In: Finkelhor D. Child sexual abuse: New research and theory. New York: Free Press, 1984: 171–187.

34. Howells K. Adult sexual interest in children: Considerations relevant to theories of etiology. In: Cook M, Howells K, eds. Adult sexual interest in children. New York: Academic Press, 1981: 55–94.

35. Quinsey VL. Men who have sex with children. In: Weisstub D, ed. Law and mental health: International perspectives. Vol. 2. New York: Pergamon, 1990.

36. Abel GG, Becker JV, Murphy WD, Falanagan B. Identifying dangerous child molesters. In: Stuart RB, ed. Violent behavior. New York: Brunner/Mazel, 1981: 116–137.

37. Freund K. Erotic preference in pedophilia. Behav Res Ther 1967; 5:209–228.

38. Freund K, Langevin R. Bisexuality in homosexual pedophilia. Arch Sex Behav 1976; 5(5):415–423.

39. Quinsey VL, Steiman CM, Bergensen SG, Holmes TF. Penile circumference, skin conduction, and ranking responses of child molesters and "normals" to sexual and nonsexual visual stimuli. Behav Ther 1975; 6:213–219.

40. Hanson R, Slater S. Sexual victimization in the history of sexual abusers: A review. Ann Sex Res 1988; 1:485–499.

41. Bard L, Carter D, Cerce D, Knight R, Rosenberg R, Schneider B. A descriptive study of rapists and child molesters: Developmental, clinical and criminal characteristics (unpublished manuscript). Bridgewater, MA, 1983.

42. Groth NA, Burgess AW. Sexual trauma in the life histories of rapists and child molesters. Victimology 1979; 4:10–16.
43. Langevin R. Sexual strands: Understanding and treating sexual anomalies in men. Hillsdale, NJ: Erlbaum Associates, 1983.
44. Pelto V. Male incest offenders and non-offenders: A comparison of early sexual history (dissertation). Ann Arbor, MI: United States International University, University Microfilms, 1981.
45. Frisbie L. Another look at sex offenders in California. Research Monograph No. 12. Sacramento: California Department of Mental Hygiene, 1969.
46. Gebhard P, Gagnon J, Pomeroy W, Christenson C. Sex offenders: An analysis of types. New York: Harper & Row, 1965.
47. Aarens M, Cameron T, Roizen J, Room R, Schneberk D, Wingard D. Alcohol and family abuse. In: Alcohol casualties and crime. Berkeley: Social Research Group, 1978: 527–574.
48. Morgan P. Alcohol and family violence: Review of the literature. Alcohol and Health Monograph 1. Washington, DC: National Institute of Alcoholism and Alcohol Abuse, Alcohol Consumption and Related Problems, 1982: 223–259.
49. Williams LM, Finkelhor D. The characteristics of incestuous fathers: A review of recent studies. In: Marshall W, Laws R, Barbaree H, eds. The handbook of sexual assault: Issues, theories and treatment of the offender. New York: Plenum, 1990.
50. Parker H, Parker S. Father-daughter sexual abuse: An emerging perspective. Am J Orthopsychiatry 1986; 56(4):531–549.
51. Abel GG, Cummingham-Rathner J, Becker JB, McHugh J. Motivating sex offenders for treatment with feedback of their psychophysiologic assessment. Paper presented at the World Congress of Behavior Therapy, Washington, DC, December, 1983.
52. Browne A, Finkelhor D. The impact of child sexual abuse: Review of the research. Psych Bull 1986; 99(1):66–77.
53. Gelinas DJ. The persisting negative effects of incest. Psychiatry 1983; 46:312–332.
54. Jehu D, Gazan M. Psychosocial adjustment of women who were sexually victimized in childhood or adolescence. Can J Community Ment Health 1983; 2:71–81.
55. Conte J, Schuerman J. Factors associated with an increased impact of child sexual abuse. Child Abuse Neglect 1987; 11:201–211.
56. Runyan D, et al. Impact of legal intervention on sexually abused children. J Pediatr 1988; 113(4):647–653.
57. Fromuth ME. The relationship of childhood sexual abuse with later psychological and sexual adjustment in a sample of college women. Child Abuse Neglect 1986; 10:5–15.
58. Peters SD. The relationship between childhood sexual victimization and adult depression among Afro-American and white women (dissertation). Los Angeles: University of California, 1984 (University Microfilms No. 84-28,555).
59. Seidner A, Calhoun KS. Childhood sexual abuse: Factors related to differential adult adjustment. Paper presented at the Second National Conference for Family Violence Researchers, Durham, NH, 1984.
60. Stein J, et al. Long-term psychological sequelae of child sexual abuse: The Los Angeles Epidemiologic Catchment Area Study. In: Wyatt G, Powell G, eds. Lasting effects of child sexual abuse. Newbury Park, CA: Sage, 1988.

61. de Young M. The sexual victimization of children. Jefferson, NC: McFarland & Co., 1982.
62. Miller J, Moeller D, Kaufman A, Divasto P, Pather D, Christy J. Recidivism among sexual assault victims. Am J Psychiatry 1978; 135:1103-1104.
63. Courtois C. The incest experience and its aftermath. Victimology 1979; 4:337-347.
64. James J, Meyerding J. Early sexual experiences and prostitution. Am J Psychiatry 1977; 134:1381-1385.
65. Silbert MN, Pines AM. Sexual child abuse as an antecedent to prostitution. Child Abuse Neglect 1981; 5:407-411.
66. Oppenheimer R, Palmer RL, Braden S. A clinical evaluation of early sexually abusive experience in adult anorexic and bulimic females: Implications for preventative work in childhood. Paper presented at the Fifth International Conference on Child Abuse and Neglect. Montreal, 1984.
67. Russell DE. The prevalence and seriousness of incestuous abuse: Stepfathers vs. biological fathers. Child Abuse Neglect 1983; 8(1):15-22.
68. Summit R. The child sexual abuse accommodation syndrome. Child Abuse Neglect 1983; 7(2):177-193.
69. Finkelhor D. The prevention of child sexual abuse: An overview of needs and problems. SIECUS Report 1984; 13(1):1-15.
70. Conte J. Research on the prevention of sexual abuse of children. Paper presented at the Second National Conference for Family Violence Researchers, Durham, NH, 1984.
71. Plummer C. Preventing sexual abuse: What in-school programs teach children. Paper presented at the Second National Conference for Family Violence Researchers, Durham, NH, 1984.
72. Finkelhor D, Strapko N. Sexual abuse prevention education: A review of evaluation studies. In: Willis D, Holder E, Rosenberg M, ed. Child abuse prevention. New York: Wiley, 1990.
73. MacFarlane K, Bulkley J. Treating child sexual abuse: An overview of current program models. In: Conte J, Shore D, eds. Social work and child sexual abuse. New York: Haworth, 1982: 69-81.
74. Sgroi S. Handbook of clinical intervention in child sexual abuse. Lexington, MA: Lexington Books, 1982.
75. Knopp FH. Retraining adult sex offenders: Methods and models. Syracuse: Safer Society Press, 1984.
76. Kelley RJ. Behavioral re-orientation of pedophiliacs: Can it be done? Clinical Psychology Review 1982; 2:387-408.
77. Saunders B, Lipovsky J, Ralston E, Sorrow R. Profile of incest perpetrators indicating treatability-Part II: Final report. Charleston, SC: Crime Victims Research and Treatment Center, 1989.
78. Simpkins L, Urand W, Bowman S, Rinck CM, DeSouza E. Predicting treatment outcome for child sexual abusers. Annals Sex Research 1990, 3:21-57.
79. Christenson K, Elers-Nielson M, Lemaine L, Sturup G. Recidivism among sexual offenders. In: Christiansen K, ed. Scandanavian Studies in Criminology, Vol. 1. London: Tavistock, 1965: 55-85.
80. Bulkley J, ed. Innovations in the prosecution of child sexual abuse cases. Washington, DC: American Bar Association, 1981.

5

Rape and Sexual Assault

JUDITH M. VON, DEAN G. KILPATRICK,
ANN W. BURGESS, AND CAROL R. HARTMAN

Contrary to popular belief, rape is not a rare event, but rather something that affects the lives of thousands of people each year. Since 1977 the rate of forcible rape has increased by 21 percent, the largest increase among all major crimes. Although most types of crime have a psychological impact on victims, sexual assault has been found to be particularly deleterious. Rape victims experience significant long-term problems in the areas of fear, anxiety, and depression, as well as difficulties in social adjustment and impaired sexual functioning. Furthermore, being the victim of rape appears to be associated with an increased risk of suicide. Sexual assault claims many indirect victims as well. For example, marriages may be jeopardized, jobs may be lost, and families and social networks disrupted when victims are forced to move themselves and their families because of the fear of further attack. In addition, the fear of being raped serves to restrict the daily mobility of many nonvictimized women.

There is general agreement that rape is the most underreported violent crime. One reason for this may be the poor treatment received by victims from the criminal justice system. Improved treatment of victims could increase victim cooperation in both reporting crimes and in providing testimony, which in turn could help prevent criminals from re-offending.

Unlike other types of crime, it is difficult to know how frequently rape occurs because of the low reporting rate for the crime. Accurate estimates of the incidence and prevalence of rape are not readily available, as the majority of rape victims do not report to police and do not seek medical attention or other forms of victim assistance.

The definition of what constitutes rape varies among states, but generally refers to forced sexual penetration of a victim by an offender who is not the victim's spouse. Some states use definitions patterned after the Federal

Bureau of Investigation (FBI) Uniform Crime Report, which limits "rape" to incidents in which the victim is female and in which only vaginal penetration has taken place. Because the legal definition of forcible rape is so restrictive, the term, sexual assault, has been used to cover a wider range of crimes, including attempted rape, indecent assault and battery, as well as sodomy. Most statutes define as illegal any type of sexual behavior with a child, regardless of the use or threat of force or victim's consent.

Data on rape and sexual assault are available at the national level from both the FBI Uniform Crime Report and the National Crime Survey. The Uniform Crime Report represents the number of forcible rapes reported annually to the police. The National Crime Survey reports victimization data gleaned from a continuing survey of representative households. A primary limitation of both data sets is the underreporting of incidents.

Victimization surveys are regarded as the best way to estimate the incidence and prevalence rate of major crimes, including rape. These surveys also provide information on the extent of underreporting, details of the attack, and information regarding medical care utilization or other forms of victim assistance. However, numerous methodological variables influence the reliability and validity of these data.

Two major theoretical models have been proposed to account for the commission of rape. The first centers on the character pathology of the offender; the second views social factors as causative. Although early research treated these two models as mutually exclusive, recent work indicates incorporating variables from both models may be necessary. One of the many strengths of recent investigations has been the extension of research from incarcerated rapists to undetected offenders. In addition, although it has been suggested that acquaintance rape and assault by strangers may require different theoretical explanations, the results of current research indicate that this may not be the case. That is, those factors found to be related to the occurrence of rape by strangers (e.g., sexual arousal in response to aggression, hostility toward women) have been found to be related to acquaintance assault as well.

Early attempts to explain the occurrence of rape focused on identifying characteristics within the victim that would render her susceptible to assault. The resulting theories are all, in varying degrees, ideologically related to a victim-blame perspective and have thus been criticized because of the lack of attention paid to offender behavior. The existing data indicate that there is no variable that consistently distinguishes rape victims from nonvictimized women.

Rape victims experience significant long-term problems in the areas of psychological functioning, social adjustment, and sexual functioning. Fear, anxiety, and depression are the most frequently identified psychological sequelae of rape. As the literature on crime victims has expanded, attention has shifted from simply describing symptoms to assessing the presence of symptom constellations consistent with major psychiatric diagnoses. Posttraumatic stress disorder (PTSD) has commonly been identified among

victims of crimes, with rape specifically acknowledged as a potential precipitant of PTSD. Other significant mental health problems associated with
sexual victimization include substance abuse and an increased risk of suicide.

Victims of rape and sexual assault require access to a comprehensive
system of services and resources. These include emergency clinical services,
crisis counseling, criminal justice system assistance, victim compensation,
and, for some victims, long-term specialized therapy.

There are many critical areas for future research; however, rape prevention remains primary. Although services to rape victims have improved
qualitatively and quantitatively during the last decade, no breakthrough has
occurred in the prevention of sexual assault. One of the implications of
eliminating or greatly reducing the rate of rape is that radical changes in the
ideology and social structure of our society must be made.

STATEMENT OF THE PROBLEM

Overview

Contrary to popular belief, rape and other forms of sexual assault are not
uncommon events. It has been estimated (1) that the population of the
United States contains more rape victims (3,750,000) than combat veterans
(2,480,544) (2). Less conservative estimates indicate that between 9,750,000
and 16,500,000 women have been victims of a completed rape at least once
in their lifetimes (3).

Since 1977 the rate of forcible rape has increased by 21 percent. That is
the largest increase among all major crimes. One researcher found that
approximately 40 percent of college women and 44 percent of women
surveyed in community studies report being victims of either attempted or
completed rape (3).

Although it has been shown that most types of crime have a psychological
impact on victims (4), sexual assault has been shown to be particularly
deleterious (5,6). A well-documented literature base (7-9) indicates that rape
victims experience significant long-term psychological problems (such as
increased fear, anxiety, and depression) as well as impaired social adjustment and sexual functioning. Further, being a victim of rape appears to be
associated with an increased risk of suicide (5,10). The results of one study
indicated that 19.2 percent of rape victims had attempted suicide, a rate 8.7
times higher than the rate for nonvictims (5). More recent data (10) indicate
that 5.2 percent of surveyed nonvictims had made a serious suicide attempt;
the corresponding rate for victims of completed rape was 19.8 percent. As
noted by one researcher (11), it is impossible to know how many victims kill
themselves as a result of crime-induced trauma.

The human suffering contained in these statistics clearly indicates that
rape and sexual assault are public health problems of major importance.
Not only are large numbers of the population affected, but available evidence suggests that the recovery rate for rape victims is slower than for

victims of other types of crime (11). Further, recovery may not be as complete as once was thought. A striking 16.5 percent of assessed rape victims were diagnosed as having crime-related posttraumatic stress disorder an average of 17 years after the assault (4).

The impact on rape victims is readily apparent. However, it must be kept in mind that sexual assault claims many indirect victims as well. For example, it is not uncommon for marriages to dissolve following sexual assault. Many victims are forced to leave jobs due to the necessity of frequent court appearances or because the fear engendered by the assault markedly impairs work performance. It is by no means uncommon for rape victims to be forced to uproot their families and relocate in order to prevent retaliation from a known attacker or the attacker's family.

Further, the fear of being raped serves to restrict the daily mobility of nonvictimized women (12–14). Results of national surveys indicate that in general, women are more fearful of crime than men (15) and that the fear of being raped is particularly salient (16).

Last, improvements in the treatment of rape victims may function as a method of crime prevention (17). There is a general consensus that rape is the most underreported violent crime and that one of the reasons for this is the poor treatment received by victims from the criminal justice system (18). Without victim cooperation in both reporting crimes and providing testimony, the criminal justice system functions ineffectively and leaves criminals free to re-offend.

Uniqueness of Rape Compared to Other Types of Violent Crime

It has been noted that when compared to other types of serious crime, rape has a number of unique characteristics. First, it is particularly difficult to know how frequently rape occurs because of the low reporting rate for this crime. Accurate estimates of the incidence and prevalence of rape are not readily available because the majority of rape victims do not report to the police, do not receive medical attention from hospitals, and do not seek help from service agencies such as rape crisis centers (19).

Second, victims of rape are often held responsible for their own assaults and assailants dismissed as not having committed a "real" offense. It is believed by many that women like to be overpowered sexually; that women say no but mean yes; and that women issue false reports regarding rape to "save face," "get even," or conceal their own responsibility for pregnancy (20). Unlike other crimes there is considerable variation in what constitutes a "real" rape (21–23). For some authorities, if the victim is of unquestioned virtue and if considerable force is employed, then the act is defined as a "real" rape. However, if a woman is forced to have sex by a man she has dated a few times and originally met in a bar, the act may not be viewed as rape (24).

Third, rape is treated distinctively in the courtroom, for example, as a property crime (22,25). Further, rules of evidence have been unique and stringent, frequently requiring signs of resistance as proof of nonconsent, or requiring third-party corroboration. An analogy has been drawn between the need to prove nonconsent and the experience of a prize fighter (26, pp. 23–24).

> To win this kind of contest, the rape victim must act like a contender for a boxing title who does not let her fans down; it must be clearly demonstrated that she did not throw the fight. Obviously, under these conditions, an absence of cuts and bruises is tellingly noted by the defense attorneys. This lack of physical evidence is used to "prove" the innocence of the accused rapist; moreover, the "proof" is reportedly "demonstrated" by maintaining that it is the woman who has the moral responsibility to prevent rape by resisting the rapist to the utmost.

Definitions

Part of the problem inherent in understanding rape and sexual assault is derived from its equivocal definition.* From a legal perspective, rape is a criminal act (24). Whereas old laws viewed rape as an act of illicit sex, more recent legislation defines rape as a type of assault. Although there are variations among states, rape as legally defined generally refers to forced sexual penetration of a victim by an offender who is not the victim's spouse. As defined by the Federal Bureau of Investigation (FBI) Uniform Crime Report (27), *forcible rape* "is the carnal knowledge of a female [obtained] forcibly and against her will. Assaults or attempts to commit rape by force or threat of force are also included; however, statutory rape (without force) and other sex offenses are excluded" (p. 13). Some states' laws that are patterned after the FBI's definition limit the application of the term rape to incidents in which the victim is female and cases in which only vaginal penetration has taken place. Specifically excluded would be incidents in which males were the victims or cases in which oral or anal penetration occurred.

Further, many statutes have a marital exclusion rule that states that the elements defining criminal sexual conduct cannot legally occur if the offender and victim are married. This marital exclusion stems from the historical legal theory that rape is actually a crime against the property of a woman's father or husband (25). If a wife is the property of her husband who has unlimited sexual access to her regardless of her consent, then the husband cannot be legally viewed as damaging his own property or of committing an illegal act of sexual aggression.

As the legal definition of forcible rape is so restrictive, *sexual assault* has been used to cover a wider range of sexual crimes including attempted rape, indecent assault and battery, as well as sodomy. Sexual assault has been

---

*Although it is recognized that men can be and are victims of sexual assault, the overwhelming majority of the existing literature is based on female victims. For purposes of this chapter, only the data pertaining to female victims are reviewed. At present, the prevalence rate for rape of males is virtually unknown; clearly this is an area that merits further study.

defined as manual, genital, or oral contact with the victim's genitalia without consent and obtained by force, threat, or fraud.

Most statutes define as illegal any type of sexual behavior with a child, irrespective of the use of force or threat of force or victim's consent. As Finkelhor (28) has noted, the general notion behind these statutory rape laws is that children are incapable of giving informed consent for sexual activity, particularly to offenders who are much older than they. Statutory rape may also be charged in those cases in which the victim is legally unable to give consent by virtue of mental deficiency, psychosis, or altered state of consciousness induced by sleep, drugs, illness, or intoxication. *Molestation* has been defined as noncoital sexual assault, and *incest* as coitus between a blood relative or caregiver (e.g., stepfather) and a youthful victim.

As public attention is directed to this area of definition, there is concurrent pressure for legal reform. Some states (e.g., Michigan, South Carolina) have re-evaluated their rape statutes and enacted new sexual assault acts that direct the court's attention to the level of violence used and away from the view of rape as a singularly sexually motivated crime (29). Also, some states have re-evaluated their laws covering marital rape (30–32) and therapist-patient sexual exploitation (33). Reformed legislation concerning rape, with its increased emphasis on force, threat of force, and coercion comes much closer to capturing the psychological essence of rape.

Problems Defining Rape

Although there is some variation among states, rape as legally defined refers to nonconsensual oral, anal, or vaginal penetration obtained through the use of force or threat of force. In practice, however, the legal definition of rape is put into operation through a restrictive social definition of rape (24,34). One of the key components of this social definition is relationship to offender. The public perception that rape involves a brutal attack by a stranger in a remote setting is firmly entrenched in our society—so much so that many individuals, including the victims themselves, do not apply the label "rape" to an assault that deviates from this commonly accepted stereotype. As a result, many women whose experiences legally qualify as rape do not view their experience as criminal. Koss (35) has termed these women "unacknowledged victims." That is, these are women whose experience meets the legal definition of rape but who do not define themselves as rape victims. Their presence testifies to the need to ask about sexual assault using behavioral descriptions, thus avoiding the subjective bias introduced by using the label "rape."

Dimensions

According to the FBI Uniform Crime Report (27), rape comprised 7 percent of the violent crime volume and 1 percent of the Crime Index total, with 87,340 offenses occurring in 1985.

Geographically, the highest rate of forcible rape was in the Western states (85 victims per 100,000 females). In descending order, the following rates were reported per region: the South (77/100,000), the Midwest (65/100,000), and the Northeast (56/100,000).

The largest numbers of forcible rapes were reported during the summer, with July registering the highest frequency. The lowest total was reported for the month of February.

The majority of rapes involve a lone victim and a lone perpetrator (36). According to the same source, 36 percent of rapes occurred in the victim's home and 58 percent of rapes took place at night between the hours of 6 P.M. and 6 A.M.

With regard to age, the victimization rate for women peaks in the 16- to 19-year-old age group. The second-highest rate occurs in the 20- to 24-year-old age group (37). According to the Bureau of Justice Statistics, the victimization rate for these two groups combined is approximately four times higher than the mean for all women.

Black women appear to be disproportionately victimized by rape (38). Furthermore, this higher rate of victimization appears consistent across all age groups. With regard to racial composition, the majority of rapes involve victims and offenders from the same racial group (39). Among reported cases of interracial rape, the majority of offenses involve black males and white females.

DATA SOURCES

In this section, we review the available data sources, providing a critique of the strengths and limitations inherent in each.

National Data Sources

Federal Bureau of Investigation (FBI)
Uniform Crime Report (UCR)
The UCR provides annual statistics based on cases that are reported to law enforcement authorities, that is, the number of forcible rapes that are reported annually to the police. The primary limitation of this data source is underreporting, as only a small percentage of forcible rapes are ever reported to the police. Government estimates indicate that for every reported rape, three to ten rapes remain unreported (40). However, other victimization surveys (4,41,42) have found that only between 5 percent and 9.5 percent of rapes were ever reported to police.

Further, of those rapes reported, some proportion are deemed unfounded by the police and hence never become part of the UCR statistics on rape. "Unfounding" refers to the process by which the police may dismiss a case (e.g., if they view the victim's report as not believable). Jurisdictions vary with regard to the policy they employ to determine if a complaint is founded or unfounded.

Another weakness of this data set is the narrowly restricted definition of the term rape (i.e., "carnal knowledge of a female forcibly and against her will"). Cases involving oral or anal penetration, male victims, or wives assaulted by their husbands are not reflected in the UCR's published statistics. Further, the FBI employs what is known as a crime hierarchy in classifying events. According to the UCR, homicide qualifies as the most serious crime, followed by rape, robbery, aggravated assault, burglary, larceny, and motor vehicle theft. Therefore, a case in which a victim was both raped and killed would be classified as a homicide.

The National Crime Survey (NCS)

The NCS reports annual victimization data based on information derived from a continuing survey of representative households (37). The NCS collects information on incidence rates for all types of crime including sexual assault occurring within a 6-month bounded interview period. The information gleaned from these surveys is then compared with the official crime statistics for that area, thus allowing an estimate of the total rate of crime, including both reported and unreported episodes.

Again, a primary limitation of this data set is the degree of underreporting. It has been noted (42) that the NCS inquires about rape in a way that decreases the likelihood that accurate information will be obtained. For example, the survey uses a "screen" question that requires the respondent to infer that it is rape that is being asked about. Further, questions regarding rape are embedded in a context of other violent crimes. Respondents who have been victimized by family or other known assailants are unlikely to perceive these experiences as criminal. Based upon their data, Koss et al. (42) recently concluded that the actual incidence rate for rape is ten to fifteen times higher than NCS estimates.

Victimization Surveys

Victimization surveys attempt to provide data on the true rate of crime. Most experts agree that these surveys are the best way to estimate the incidence and prevalence rate of major crimes, including rape (36,43,44). These surveys involve interviewing a sample of the general population. Those who disclose having been victimized are then questioned regarding whether or not they reported the assault as well as details of the attack. In some surveys, victims are asked whether they sought medical care or help from victim service agencies. Thus information obtained from these surveys provides valuable data about incidence and prevalence as well as the apparent extent of underreporting. Nonetheless, as these surveys never identify *all* victims, obtained victimization rates are almost always an underestimate of true incidence and prevalence (1).

Factors Influencing the Reliability and Validity
of Data Obtained in Victimization Surveys

Numerous methodological variables influence the reliability and validity of victimization survey data (36,44–46). For example, Skogan's review (36, p. 11) identifies four major errors in the retrospective measurement of victimization: (1) ignorance of events, (2) forgetting (or not telling), (3) inaccuracy or incomplete recall (or lying), and (4) differential interview productivity.

The first error, *ignorance of events*, was primarily a problem of earlier surveys that asked one respondent per household about crimes that had occurred involving all household members. Obviously, if that respondent lacked knowledge of a crime happening to another household member, the respondent would be unable to report it to the survey. Almost all recent surveys deal with this problem by asking respondents only about crimes that have happened to them personally.

The second error, *forgetting or not telling*, has an important impact on all victimization studies. As Skogan (36) notes, in practice, it is usually impossible to distinguish between nondisclosure of incidents due to forgetting or due to not telling. In any case, a number of reverse-records-check studies (47–50) provide convincing proof that not all incidents reported by victims to police are subsequently remembered and disclosed to interviewers in victimization studies. It is also clear that recall and/or disclosure of a victimization experience appears to decline as a function of the length of time since the experience occurred. Moreover, there is also evidence that recall/disclosure varies as a function of the type of incident and the demand characteristics of the survey. Demand characteristics refer to the respondent's perception of the interviewer's expectations. Both Turner (49) and Catlin and Murray (47) found that personal assaults committed by strangers were more likely to be recalled and disclosed than those committed by assailants known by the victim. Some evidence suggests that "serious" incidents are no more likely to be remembered/disclosed than less serious ones (48,51,52). With respect to demand characteristics, pretests for the National Crime Survey found that the number of incidents recalled/disclosed decreased if a detailed incident report was completed after each disclosure instead of asking all screening questions prior to obtaining incident reports.

A major limitation of all reverse-records-check studies conducted to date is that they deal only with incidents that have first been reported to police. Thus it is difficult to determine whether recall/disclosure of the nonreported incidents is similar to that of reported incidents. Obviously, an incident that is not recalled and disclosed will deflate estimates of incidence and prevalence.

The third error, *inaccuracy or incomplete recall*, refers to respondents remembering and disclosing an incident but providing inaccurate information about one or more details of the incident. Most of the emphasis in studies of this type of error has focused upon respondents' difficulties in correctly identifying exactly when the incident occurred in time. Temporal telescoping is the term used to describe a tendency for people to remember an event but place it at the wrong point in time. Forward telescoping occurs when an event is remembered as occurring closer to the present than when it actually occurred, and backward telescoping is when an event is remembered as occurring more distant in time from the present than it actually occurred. Forward telescoping is generally felt to be more prevalent and to pose a particularly great problem for incidence studies. Obviously, any tendency for individuals to recall and disclose incidents occurring prior to the reference period as having occurred during the reference period will inflate estimates of incidence during that period.

As Skogan (36) notes, it is possible to minimize the problem of telescoping by (1) reducing the length of the reference period (time period from present), and (2) "bounding" the interview. The latter term refers to a procedure of collecting information about victimization in a panel design of two or more interviews. Victimization information collected during the first interview is ignored since it is thought to be inflated by forward telescoping. Information about victimization occurring in the period *between* the two interviews is used to provide incidence estimates.

The National Crime Survey uses a panel-bounded interview design in which the reference period is the past six months. This reference period was a compromise. Obviously, problems with recall and telescoping diminish if the reference period is short and would be shortest if the reference period was "the day prior to the interview." However, crimes are relatively rare events, so sample sizes must be increased if the reference period length is decreased to generate sufficient numbers of cases to study. Even with a six-month reference period, the National Crime Survey has a sample size of about 58,000 households and interviews about 132,000 respondents every six months (53).

Use of short reference periods and bounded interviews produces more accurate estimates of the incidence of victimization experiences of interest. Based on comparisons of incidence rates from bounded and unbounded interviews in the National Crime Survey, it appears that unbounded interviews produce rates about one-third higher than those obtained from bounded interviews. However, using short reference periods and bounded interviews can provide *no* information about any victimization experiences that occurred prior to the bounded interview. Thus the National Crime Survey approach is incapable of providing information about lifetime prevalence of victimization. If one is interested in lifetime prevalence, there is no alternative but to extend the reference period to the respondent's entire lifetime and to use an unbounded interview. Doing so increases telescoping and inaccuracy of recall, facts that the researcher must understand and acknowledge. However, short of beginning a lifelong panel design victimization survey at a child's birth, it is difficult to determine any better way than an unbounded retrospective study to investigate lifetime prevalence of victimization.

The fourth error described by Skogan (36) is *differential productivity* of respondents. Briefly, this refers to the tendency for more highly educated respondents to be more at ease in interview situations, to be more cooperative, and to generally report more victimization experiences to interviewers. As Skogan discusses, results of the National Crime Survey as well as a number of similar surveys conducted in other countries indicate that disclosures of incidents of assaultive violence increase as a function of the educational status of respondents. For example, examination of data from the 1976 National Crime Survey indicated that college-educated respondents disclosed approximately three times as many incidents of assaultive violence as respondents who had only attended or completed elementary school. Since most experts believe that people with lower educational and socioeconomic status actually experience the bulk of criminal victimization, these findings are counterintuitive and perplexing. Several possible explanations for such findings have been proposed. Some suggest that crime is more salient to well-educated respondents because it is less a part of their everyday lives. Others state that well-educated respondents differ only in their increased ability to recall and disclose less serious types of assault, such as attempted crimes (48). Others suggest that such findings are primarily an artifact of well-educated respondents' greater familiarity with and cooperation in interview situations (36,54). It is also possible that conventional wisdom is wrong and that better educated people actually do experience more victimization than less well-educated ones. In any case, evidence is relatively clear that the tendency for well-educated respondents to disclose more victimization experiences than those who are less well-educated may account for some differences in prevalence of rape and sexual assault reported by various studies. In fact, studies that have reported highest lifetime prevalence of sexual assault have had relatively high percentages of college-educated respondents in their samples (3,55).

Need to Improve Data Sources

The clear impact of the previously discussed definitional issues on the rates obtained in incidence and prevalence studies is twofold. First, how sexual assault is operationally defined and screened for by researchers will have a profound impact on the incidence and prevalence figures obtained.

Second, as several experts have noted (3,56,57), it is of vital importance to ask about specific experiences defined in behavioral terms rather than asking about having been raped, sexually assaulted, or attacked. (For example, "Have you ever been forced to have sexual intercourse when you did not want to?" or "Have you ever had sexual intercourse when you did not want to because a man threatened or physically forced you?" as opposed to "Have you ever been raped?") Failure to use behavioral terms will likely result in a considerable underestimate of incidence and prevalence. Thus the number of sexual assault and rape incidents both detected and reported depends upon the victims' and the authorities' (e.g., police, researcher's) perception of what occurred. That is, a woman may not conceptualize her experience as rape. Alternatively, the police or prosecutor may dismiss any complaint they believe is "unfounded."

The social/psychological process involved in getting sexual assault and rape incidents recorded is contained in an elaboration of the steps necessary for police to become aware of a crime incident (48). (Note: the same steps would be involved in a researcher's detection of the same events.) First, victims must *perceive* the event in question to have occurred. Second, they must recognize and *classify* the event as belonging to a category of illegal activities. Third, they must decide whether or not to *disclose* it. According to Sparks and his colleagues (48), the fourth step in this process is a *redefinition* on the part of the police (or researcher) who decides in questioning whether the disclosed events meet the definition of the illegal act. Only if the police (or researcher) defines the event as the type they are interested in does the fifth step, *recording* of the incident, occur.

As illustrated by this conceptual model, the process of definition is important at two key steps in the recording process: first, at the respondent's or victim's level and second, at the inquirer's level. If there is substantial disagreement, then the groundwork is set for considerable underrepresentation in victimization surveys.

CAUSES AND RISK FACTORS

Research on Sexual Offenders

Early attempts to explain male involvement in sexual aggression resulted in the development of two major theoretical models. The first model focused on the individual psychopathology of the offender and resulted in numerous studies in which rapists were compared to nonrapists on a variety of psychological tests (58). Attempts to find empirical support for this model have been unsuccessful. For example, Perdue and Lester (59) found no significant differences between the Rorschach responses of rapists and prisoners who had committed violent, nonsexual crimes. Studies examining other psychological test results such as the Minnesota Multiphasic Personality Inventory (MMPI) (60) have found that rapists do manifest elevations on Scale 4 (Psychopathic Deviate), but do not typically differ from other criminal groups on this scale.

The greatest limitation inherent in research examining the characteristics of rapists has been the nonrepresentativeness of the samples employed. Samples of rapists studied have generally been obtained from correctional or other institutional settings such as psychiatric facilities. As the percentage of rapes reported and convicted is extremely small and as it has been shown that convicted rapists differ from those unapprehended (58,61), the generalizability of these data is limited.

Scully and Marolla (62) argue that rape has become a "medicalized" social problem. They suggest that the notion of rape as a nonutilitarian act committed by a few "sick" men is too limited a view of sexual violence because it excludes culture and social structure as predisposing factors. Scully and Marolla's analysis of 114 incarcerated rapists revealed that rapists used sexual violence as a method of revenge and/or punishment, a means of gaining access to unwilling or unavailable women, a bonus added to burglary or robbery, a recreational activity, and a form of impersonal sex that gained the offender power over his victims.

In contrast to the psychopathology model discussed above, the social control/social conflict model maintains that perpetrators adhere to a belief system that allows them to both engage in and justify rape. This system is believed to be the result of the influence of a society that legitimizes violence (of which sexual aggression is one form) against women. In this model, sexual aggression against females is not the result of any diagnosable, individual pathology, but rather is due to acceptance of societal attitudes that foster male dominance and dehumanize females, making them simply objects. The results of numerous studies (63) have supported this model by showing a relationship between certain attitudes (e.g., acceptance of rape myths, sex role stereotyping) and various measures of aggression. For example, Koss, Leonard, Beezly, and Oros (64) found that sexually aggressive men could be differentiated from nonaggressive males on the basis of measures reflecting rape-supportive attitudes.

Early research tended to treat these two models as if they were mutually exclusive. However, newer work suggests that incorporating variables from both models may be requisite. Rapaport and Burkhart (65) provide support for characterological mediation of sexual aggression. That is, they found that nonincarcerated sexually aggressive males displayed both characterological deficits (e.g., irresponsibility and poor socialization) and adherence to an attitudinal system that perceives women as adversaries and that legitimizes the use of aggression, particularly in a sexual situation.

One of the many strengths of recent investigations (e.g., 64,65) has been the extension of research to undetected offenders. Additional gains have been made by examining the causes of male sexual aggression against women from an interactionist perspective. For example, Barlow and associates (66,67) examined the interrelation between four variables of sexual functioning including both deviant and appropriate sexual arousal, heterosocial skills, and gender-role behavior. With respect to acknowledged sex offenders (i.e., rapists, child molesters), it has been asserted that poor social skills may be one of multiple etiological factors. Proponents of this social deficit model have argued that these offenders lack the skills and behavior needed to adequately engage in social interactions with women. Initial explorations (68,69) as well as more methodologically sound studies (70) have provided support for this view.

Most recently, attempts to explain male sexual aggression have resulted in complex integrative and multidimensional theorizing (71,72). Stimulated by Finkelhor's work on child abusers (73), these authors have examined the interaction between such variables as internal motivation, deviant sexual arousal, and reduction of internal and external inhibition of aggression. In general, the results of these studies suggest a synergistic process. For example, Koss and Dinero (72) concluded that there appeared to be a "developmental sequence for sexual aggression in which early experiences and psychological characteristics establish preconditions for sexual violence" (p. 16). These preconditions were then dependent upon current environmental factors for sexual aggression to occur.

Although it has been suggested that acquaintance rape and stranger assault may require different theoretical explanations (74,75), the results of current research (71) indicate that this may not be the case. That is, those factors found to be related to the occurrence of stranger rape (e.g., sexual arousal in response to aggression, hostility toward women) have been found to be related to acquaintance assault as well.

Victim Characteristics

Early attempts to explain the occurrence of rape focused on identifying characteristics within the victim that would render her susceptible to assault. Three models have been proposed: victim precipitation, social control, and situational blame. These models are presented here to acquaint the reader with them. However, it should be clear to the reader that there are no empirical data to support these models and that all these models, to varying degrees, are ideologically related to a victim-blame perspective.

Victim Precipitation

This model, first proposed by Amir (76), generally posits that specific behaviors or personality characteristics heighten susceptibility to rape. Amir based his theoretical position on the observation from police records that rape victims were often described as having a "bad reputation," and thus could be partially held responsible for the assault. Another adherent of this line of reasoning, Kanin (77), has argued that assailants often attributed their behavior to some aspect of the woman's appearance and/or demeanor (e.g., "she dressed like that").

In a variation of this general model (sometimes referred to as a vulnerability model of rape), Selkin (78) examined personality differences between "rape resisters" (i.e., attempted rape victims) and rape victims, and found that resisters scored higher on certain measures such as dominance and social pressure. From this he concluded that victims had a greater likelihood of being raped because of such characteristics as passivity.

It should be noted that empirical support for this model is extremely limited. Further, these findings have been criticized on several grounds. Most notably, Koss and Harvey (79, p. 20) have argued that "police judgments of reputation and a rapist's rationale for raping are not unbiased information." Further, unbiased sampling from rape victims, attempted rape victims, victims of sexual coercion, and nonvictimized women revealed no differences in personality characteristics as measured by the California Psychological Inventory (35).

Social Control

The social control model posits that the victims' belief system increases their vulnerability to assault. Evidence for this model has generally come from studies examining acceptance of rape myths (e.g., "the victim really wanted it") among various groups including the general public, police, rape counselors, and rapists (20,80,81). The only study to date that has directly examined victim adherence to such a belief system found no support for this hypothesis. Koss (35) compared rape victims and nonvictimized females on seven attitudinal variables including acceptance of sexual aggression, attitudes toward female sexuality, rejection of rape myths, unacceptability of aggression, heterosexual relationships as game playing, rape attitudes, and attitudes toward women, and found no significant differences between groups. More importantly, Koss hypothesized that among sexually victimized women, degree of acceptance of rape-supportive beliefs may be related to whether a woman labels her assault as rape. However, she found no significant differences between acknowledged and unacknowledged victims with regard to acceptance of rape myths.

Situational Blame Model

This model contends that rape is more likely to occur in particular environmental contexts and subsequent to particular victim/perpetrator behaviors. Support for this model has generally come from studies of rape avoidance in which comparisons were made between resistance strategies employed by women who avoided rape and those who failed to avoid rape. The evidence to date suggests that differences in the ability to avoid rape are the result of strategies utilized as opposed to demographic or background variables. For example, Bart (82) demonstrated that women were more likely to avoid rape if they were attacked by strangers, were outside any building, employed multiple resistance strategies (e.g., screaming and physically struggling), and were most concerned with not being raped as opposed to being otherwise physically harmed. Alternatively, women were more likely to be raped if they were assaulted at home, knew their assailants (especially if they had had a prior sexual relationship), employed talking as a resistance strategy, and were primarily concerned with avoiding death or mutilation.

To summarize, there are no findings to date that consistently distinguish rape victims from nonvictimized women on either attitudinal or personality variables. Those studies finding some differences have been retrospective in nature (78). Further, prevalence rates alone would argue against over-reliance on a pathological or "victim precipitation" model. Whereas rape avoidance studies suggest possible preventive strategies (and are important in that regard), their contribution to an understanding of acquaintance rape has been criticized because of the lack of attention paid to offender behaviors (79).

Societal Factors

In the 1970s, feminists attempted to raise the awareness of others that the act of rape and the victim's response were strongly linked to the social discrimination and oppression surrounding the sex role ascribed to women. Traditional socialization patterns, argued feminists, encourage males to associate power, strength, and dominance with masculinity, while femininity is associated with passivity, submission, weakness, and inferiority. As Weis and Borges (83) note, socialization prepares women to be "legitimate" victims. Feminists emphasized that rape served the social control function of keeping women "in their place" (12,25,84). They argued that the end result is that social practices and beliefs which legitimize sexual aggression against women do so as a way of maintaining the inequitable distribution of power in our society.

Empirical studies have shown that violence and sex are intertwined in a multiplicity of ways in our society even in supposedly normal males. It has been suggested that rape exists on a continuum with what many people regard as "normal" heterosexuality. Evidence for this position has come from studies demonstrating a proclivity to rape among college-age males (85). In a review of the literature examining sexual aggression among acquaintances, Burkhart and Stanton (34, p. 7) concluded that "sexual aggression, at least by count, is normative; it is embedded in the social structure of courtship." Studies examining non-college-based samples have generally come to the same conclusion (57).

OUTCOMES

Effects of Victimization

The psychological sequelae of rape have been well documented, starting with clinical studies (86,87) and advancing to controlled studies (8,9). In particular, four categories of postrape reactions have been empirically examined, including fear and anxiety (88,89), depression (90,91), sexual dysfunction (92–94), and impairment in social functioning (95–97).

As the literature on crime victims has expanded, there has been a shift from simply describing symptoms to assessing the presence of symptom constellations consistent with major psychiatric diagnoses. Posttraumatic stress disorder (PTSD) (98) has been one diagnosis that has commonly been identified among victims of crime (1,9,10). With regard to sexual assault, rape has been specifically acknowledged as a potential precipitant of PTSD (98). Briefly stated, PTSD represents a characteristic set of symptoms that result from exposure to a psychologically traumatic event. Such trauma can include natural (e.g., earthquake, floods), accidental (e.g., airplane/car accidents), or deliberate, man-made disasters (e.g., rape, concentration camps). The hallmark symptoms of PTSD include (1) a reexperiencing of the event through persistent, intrusive, and distressing recollections; (2) mood disturbances including diminished responsiveness, loss of interest or feelings of estrangement; and (3) increased arousal (e.g., exaggerated startle response, hypervigilance) and behavioral avoidance of stimuli that resemble the traumatic event. Virtually all of the symptoms that define PTSD have been documented in victims of rape (50,96,97,99).

Limited data exist on the proportion of rape victims who develop PTSD. However, Kilpatrick, Saunders, Veronen, Best, and Von (4) found that approximately 28 percent of assessed crime victims subsequently developed PTSD. Among rape victims, 57 percent developed PTSD sometime following the assault, and approximately 17 percent still had PTSD when assessed an average of 17 years after the rape. Recent data (6) indicate that development of PTSD is positively associated with three variables. These variables include being the victim of a completed rape, sustaining a physical injury, and cognitive appraisal of life threat (i.e., believing that you would be killed or seriously harmed during commission of a crime). Kilpatrick et al. (6) found that victims possessing all three of these variables were 8.5 times more likely to develop PTSD.

Relationship Between Criminal Victimization and the Development of Significant Mental Health Problems

Recently conducted research indicates that a history of criminal victimization significantly increases the likelihood of current mental health problems, including social phobia, sexual dysfunction, major depression, and obsessive compulsive disorders (10). Similarly, two epidemiological studies of catchment areas located in Los Angeles, California (100), and Durham, North Carolina (101), found that when compared to nonvictims, sexual assault victims were more likely to report a lifetime history of major depression, dysthymic disorder, anxiety disorder, and substance abuse.

Suicide

Available evidence suggests that a history of sexual assault is associated with an increased risk of suicide. Kilpatrick et al. (5) found that 19 percent of surveyed rape victims had attempted suicide. Alternatively, only 2.2 percent of nonvictims had made an attempt. Similar data have been reported by Resick (11) who found that 17 percent of rape victims seeking treatment reported making a suicide attempt. Kilpatrick et al. (10) found that whereas approximately 17 percent of female nonvictims had ever seriously contemplated suicide, 37 percent of rape victims had done so. With regard to actual attempts, only 5.2 percent of nonvictims had made a serious suicide attempt; however, the rate for completed-rape victims was 19.8 percent.

INTERVENTIONS

Victims of rape and sexual assault require a comprehensive system of
services and resources; victims report wanting and needing these services.
Although we need to know a great deal more about the treatment of victims
of rape and sexual assault, the following measures can be recommended as
effective interventions.

Crisis Services

Hotline
A twenty-four hour rape hotline should be staffed by trained personnel who
can provide assistance, information, and referrals for acute care, crisis and
long-term counseling, criminal justice assistance, and additional needed
services.

Victim Accompaniment
Trained staff should be available to accompany victims to the hospital
following an assault. Such services increase the likelihood that a rape victim
will utilize medical care (79). Accompaniment to the hospital can also serve
the much needed function of insuring that rape victims are adequately
informed regarding hospital procedures (including procedures for the collection of evidence). As many initial police interviews are conducted at the
hospital, accompaniment provides trained advocates who can help victims
make informed choices regarding prosecution.

Crisis Counseling
Crisis counseling is generally provided by mental health workers after the
emergency services have been completed. The basic assumptions underlying this type of intervention include: (1) the rape represents a crisis in
the victim's life; (2) the victim is regarded as "normal" or functioning
adequately prior to the external stressful event; (3) crisis intervention
aims to return the victim to pre-rape level of functioning as quickly as
possible. The crisis model is issue-oriented treatment designed to ameliorate symptoms of anxiety, fear, depression, loss of control, and decreased
assertiveness (102).

This model of crisis intervention, first used by paraprofessionals at rape
crisis centers in the early 1970s, includes a strong advocacy framework (103).
Most crisis counseling efforts have followed, in modified form, this combination of outreach, emergency care, and advocacy assistance programming.
The objective of the model is to validate the crisis nature of the event, review
the details of the rape, and focus on issues raised by the crisis. This focus is
on the assault and its aftermath with an emphasis on (1) assisting the person
to achieve mastery over the life-threatening anxiety created by the rape,
(2) identifying a supportive social network, and (3) seeking self-enhancing

ways of solving problems related to the rape and the subsequent events that occur (i.e., criminal investigations, court procedures).

Mental Health Services for Victims

Some victims will require short-term counseling following a sexual assault. Others may be in need of longer term therapy from a skilled therapist, experienced in working with victims of sexual assault. A number of effective treatment procedures have been developed to target specific rape-induced symptomatology. They include Stress Innoculation Training (24,104) to aid in the reduction of fear and anxiety, a cognitive-behavioral approach for the alleviation of depression (105), and techniques developed to address rape-related sexual dysfunction (93). For excellent discussions of treatment of victims whose assaults did not occur in the recent past, the reader is referred to Koss and Harvey (79) and Ochberg (106).

Family Intervention

Emphasis in the literature has been primarily on the victim's response to the rape and less attention has been paid to the impact of the rape on the family and community (107,108). Nevertheless, members of the victim's social network will experience stress, particularly in those cases of brutalizing rapes where victims have come close to death. As family members hear of the victimization they begin to re-create the victim's experience in their own minds. This process can trigger a posttrauma response in the victim and the family depending on how this information is received, stored, and regulated. Barlow and Wolfe (109) have suggested that unless intervention is provided, the family might play a role through this mechanism in the maintenance of anxiety.

Criminal Justice Services

Following crisis care, the victim may be referred for counseling and/or victim services within the criminal justice system. When a rape is reported to police, there is the possibility that a suspect can be identified and an arrest made. When an arrest is made, a victim automatically becomes involved in the criminal justice system. Services that can be useful during this time period and that can be provided by the victim-witness staff of the prosecutor's office include keeping the victim informed of the charges filed and any bail considerations. Prior to any court appearance, the victim is provided an orientation to the courthouse and the courtroom, and a description of what to expect in a hearing or a trial. After trial, many states allow the victim to be involved in the sentencing process by providing a victim-impact statement. After sentencing, the victim needs to be kept informed about probation revocation hearings, parole hearings, escapes, appeals, and other issues related to the criminal justice system.

Victim Compensation Programs

Victim compensation programs are an important part of comprehensive services. The Victims of Crime Act of 1984 requires that in order to receive federal funds states must offer mental health counseling to victims. Each state must decide how to implement this requirement. At this stage in the development of victim services, there are many prototypes of programs, services, and treatments, but no comprehensive model or structure for how the various components should be organized or related to one another.

Further Research

There are many critical areas for further research but none as great as the area of rape prevention. Services to rape victims have increased in quantity and improved in quality in the last decade, but Swift (110) observes that no breakthrough has been achieved in preventing sexual assault. In fact, reported rates of these crimes keep increasing.

A goal of primary intervention is to eliminate rape from society. If rape is fostered by certain social structures and beliefs, preventive efforts must focus on altering those beliefs. There are both optimistic and pessimistic implications of this interpretation. The encouraging implication is that high rates of rape are not inevitable. It is possible for a society to be rape-free, or at least have a very low rape rate (111). The discouraging implication is that to eliminate rape, one would have to make radical changes in the ideology and social structure of our society.

Strategies to prevent rape vary along two dimensions: (1) whether the strategy aims to change individual behavior or societal norms, beliefs, and values; and (2) whether the strategy targets the victim or the perpetrator. At the individual level, preventive strategies could focus on teaching individual women to avoid rape; at a societal level, preventive strategies could seek to change socialization patterns for male and female children and improve relevant service systems (e.g., criminal justice, mental health) for their symbolic and deterrent effect. Traditionally, individual-level prevention efforts have focused on altering the victim's behavior, for example, telling her not to go out alone at night and not to leave windows open or cars unlocked. Little has been done to encourage men to stop their behavior. Swift (112) suggested that the early identification and treatment of sexually victimized boys might arrest the development of abusing behaviors. The linking of childhood sexual abuse and victimizing behaviors has been noted in adult sex offenders (113–115).

There needs to be more research in the area of treatment of the rape victim. Interventions must be compatible with the victim's needs if they are to be effective in preventing or treating distressing psychological symptoms. The important work of Horowitz (116) addresses part of this question. He studied whether intrusive and repetitive thoughts after experimental stress are characteristic of certain individuals or whether such thoughts represent a more widespread stress response. He concluded that the "symptoms" of repetitive imagery, thoughts, sounds, and feelings are part of a general stress response that can be understood by a model of information processing. The continued manifestation of intrusive imagery indicates that the victim, overwhelmed with new information, is attempting to place important information in storage, the first step being recent memory. It is relegated to long-term memory only when more important information takes its place. Based on Horowitz's propositions, symptoms can now be understood as part of a process of cognitive reorganization. Therapeutic techniques that address this process hold promise for victims.

Another new area of research is the psychobiology of posttraumatic stress, that is, how victims deal with the stored memory of the trauma itself. Bessel van der Kolk and colleagues (117), using a prototype of an animal model of inescapable shock, proposed that the diminished motivation, decline in social and occupational functioning, and global constriction seen in posttrauma reactions result from decreased levels of a chemical neurotransmitter, a hyponoradrenergic state. In discussing the intrusive reexperience and sleep disturbance phenomena, they suggest that long-term augmentation of the locus ceruleus pathways following trauma may underlie the recollections and nightmares that plague patients. The more we understand about posttraumatic stress in terms of its psychobiological characteristics, and in terms of the social context in which recovery takes place (or fails to), the more information we will have in ultimately designing effective interventions.

Research on victims and victimizers needs to take place within the continued investigation of the social context that gives rise to violence and sex crimes. The fact that most rapists are male means that social forces operating through family and community social networks need to be evaluated for their contribution to the support of violent and exploitative behaviors. The effects of violent media portrayals and pornography also need to be investigated.

Finally, attention must be turned to the prevention of sexual aggression among acquaintances. At present, the majority of intervention programs focus on stranger rape; but given the incidence rates, this effort should be redirected. Efforts should be made to target those at risk for both perpetrating and suffering this form of victimization before they begin dating. If Burt (20, p. 229) is correct in stating that "the task of preventing rape is tantamount to revamping a significant portion of our social values," then the time to begin is now.

ANNOTATED BIBLIOGRAPHY

The literature on rape and sexual assault has proliferated rapidly over the past decade. Where journal articles at first sufficed, books now abound within specialty areas. In addition to the references cited for this chapter, we wish to cite three bibliographies as additional resources:

Chappel D, Geis G, Forgarty F. Forcible rape: Bibliography. J Criminal Law Criminology 1974; 65:248–263.

Walker MJ. Toward the prevention of rape: A bibliography (partially annotated). Report No. 27, mimeographed. University, AL: Center for Correctional Psychology, Department of Psychology, University of Alabama, 1975.

White R, Terrell A. Victim services bibliography: An annotation by subject. Washington, DC: National Organization for Victim Assistance, 1984.

Texts

Rape Victims and Their Care

Burgess AW, Holmstrom LL. Rape: Crisis and recovery. West Newton, MA: Awab, Inc., 1986.

> This book reports on a clinical study on 109 child, adolescent, and adult rape victims who entered a large urban hospital's emergency department over a one-year period with the chief complaint, "I've been raped." The crisis counseling technique used during the emergency period includes an admission interview and short-term follow-up by home visit, telephone, and/or accompanying the victim to court. Legal issues and procedures are covered; special populations are discussed. A follow-up interview four to six years later helps to identify the long-term issues and implications for victim therapy.

Koss MP, Harvey MR. The rape victim: Clinical and community approaches to treatment. Lexington, MA: Stephen Greene Press, 1987.

> This book provides information on needed services for rape victims as well as information relevant to assessing the quality and comprehensiveness of existing local services. In addition, a whole chapter is devoted to the development of the rape crisis center movement with a detailed study of nine exemplary rape crisis centers. The chapter on prevention of sexual assault is particularly recommended.

McCombie SL, ed. The rape crisis intervention handbook: A guide for care. New York: Plenum, 1980.

> This edited volume includes sections on the myths and realities of rape, the hospital emergency room, the legal system, rape law and the judicial process, psychological overview of rape trauma, psychological intervention, and special considerations (the child victim, and the interactions between the male counselor and female rape victim).

Ochberg F, ed. Post-traumatic therapy and victims of violence. Washington, DC: American Psychiatric Association, 1988.

> This edited volume contains chapters on the therapy of persons experiencing various types of traumatic events, of which rape trauma is one type.

Rodabaugh BJ, Austin M. Sexual assault: A guide for community action. New York: Garland STPM Press, 1981.

> This book contains several extremely helpful chapters geared to the needs of specific agencies and service providers. For example, there is a chapter on planning community programs, an appendix listing the recommendations of a citizens advisory council on rape, as well as chapters relevant to law enforcement agencies and medical service providers. The suggestions contained in this book are detailed enough to be readily implemented.

Police and Prosecution

Hazelwood RR, ed. Rape investigation. New York: Elsevier, 1986.

> This edited volume contains chapters on the latest technique in evidence collection and analysis written by special agents of the FBI crime analysis units. Contributed chapters by physicians, nurses, prosecutors, and psychologists are also included.

Victims rights. Pepperdine Law Review 1984;11 (August).

> The victims' rights movement has only recently gained national attention. Advances in victims' rights are seen in legislation on the federal and state levels and in various victim support groups.

Rowland J. The ultimate violation. New York: Doubleday & Co., 1985.

> A former California prosecutor discusses how the use of expert testimony to describe rape trauma syndrome can help juries understand what, in fact, the victim has experienced. Based on her courtroom experiences, she details four separate cases and the use of expert testimony in each case.

Sexual Violence

Prentky RA, Quinsey VL. Human sexual aggression, vol. 528. New York: Annals of the New York Academy of Sciences, 1988.

> This book is a compilation of research papers on sexual aggression and is organized into sections on psychological and typological issues, social and cross-cultural issues, biological issues, treatment and prevention, victim issues, and social policy.

REFERENCES

1. Kilpatrick DG, Veronen LJ, Best CL. Factors predicting psychological distress among rape victims. In: Figley CR, ed. Trauma and its wake. New York: Brunner/Mazel, 1985: 113–141.
2. Veterans Administration. Myths and realities: A study of attitudes toward Vietnam era veterans. Washington, DC: Harris and Associates, 1980.
3. Koss MP. The scope of rape: Implications for the clinical treatment of victims. Clin Psychol 1983; 36(4):88–91.
4. Kilpatrick DG, Saunders BE, Veronen LJ, Best CL, Von JM. Criminal victimization: Lifetime prevalence, reporting to police, and psychological impact. Crime Delinquency 1987; 33:468–478.
5. Kilpatrick DG, Best CL, Veronen LJ, Amick AE, Villeponteaux LA, Ruff GA. Mental health correlates of criminal victimization: A random community survey. J Consult Clin Psychology 1985; 53:866–873.
6. Kilpatrick DG, Saunders BE, Amick-McMullan A, Best CL, Veronen LJ, Resnick HS. Victim and crime factors associated with the development of crime-related Post-traumatic Stress Disorder. Behavior Therapy 1989; 20:199–214.
7. Ellis EM. A review of empirical rape research: Victim reactions and response to treatment. Clin Psych Rev 1983; 3:473–490.
8. Holmes MR, St. Lawrence JB. Treatment of rape-induced trauma: Proposed behavioral conceptualization and review of the literature. Clin Psych Rev 1983; 3:417–433.
9. Steketee G, Foa EB. Rape-victims: Post-traumatic stress responses and their treatment: A review of the literature. J Anxiety Disorders 1987; 1:69–86.
10. Kilpatrick DG, Veronen LJ, Saunders BE, Best CL, Amick-McMullan A, Paduhovich J. The psychological impact of crime: A study of randomly surveyed crime victims. National Institute of Justice, Grant No. 84-IJ-CX-0039, Final report, 1987.
11. Resick PA. Psychological effects of victimization: Implications for the criminal justice system. Crime Delinquency 1987; 33(4):468–478.

12. Griffin S. Rape: The all-American crime. Ramparts, September, 1971.
13. Gordon MT, Heath L. The news business, crime and fear. In: Lewis DA, ed. Reactions to crime. Beverly Hills, CA: Sage, 1981.
14. Warr M. Fear of rape among urban women. Social Problems 1985; 32(3):238–250.
15. Stinchcombe AL, Adams R, Heimer CA, Scheppele KL, Smith TW, Taylor DG. Crime and punishment: Changing attitudes and America. San Francisco, CA: Jossey-Bass, 1980.
16. Riger S, Gordon M. The fear of rape: A study in social control. J Social Issues 1981; 37(4):71–92.
17. Kilpatrick DG, Otto RK. Constitutionally guaranteed participation in criminal proceedings for victims: Potential effects on psychological functioning. Wayne Law Review 1987; 34(1):7–28.
18. Kidd RF, Chayet EF. Why victims fail to report? The psychology of criminal victimization. J Social Issues 1984; 40:34–50.
19. Kilpatrick DG, Best CL, Veronen LJ. Rape victims: Have we studied the tip of the iceberg? Paper presented at the meeting of the American Psychological Association, Anaheim, CA, August 1983.
20. Burt MR. Cultural myths and supports for rape. J Personality Social Psych 1980; 38:217.
21. Holmstrom LL, Burgess AW. The victim of rape: Institutional reactions. New York: Wiley, 1978. New Brunswick, NJ: Transaction, 1983.
22. Sanders WB, ed. Rape and women's identity. Beverly Hills, CA: Sage, 1980.
23. Williams LS. The classic rape: When do victims report? Social Problems 1984; 31(4):460–467.
24. Veronen LJ, Kilpatrick DG. Stress management for rape victims. In: Meichenbaum D, Jaremko ME, eds. Stress reduction and prevention. New York: Plenum, 1983: 341–373.
25. Brownmiller S. Against our will: Men, women and rape. New York: Simon and Schuster, 1975.
26. Schwendinger JR, Schwendinger H. Rape and inequality. Beverly Hills, CA: Sage, 1983.
27. Federal Bureau of Investigation. Crime in the United States: Uniform crime reports. Washington, DC: US Dept. of Justice, 1986.
28. Finkelhor D. What's wrong with sex between adults and children: Ethics and the problem of sexual abuse. Am J Orthopsychiatry 1979; 49(4):692–697.
29. Cobb KA, Schauer NR. Michigan's criminal sexual assault law. In: Chappel D, Geis R, Geis G, eds. Forcible rape: The crime, the victim, and the offender. New York: Columbia University Press, 1977: 170–188.
30. Schulman J. The marital rape exemption. National Center on Women and Family Law Newsletter 1980; 1:6–8.
31. Russell DEH, ed. Rape in marriage. New York: Macmillan, 1982.
32. Finklehor D, Yllo K. License to rape: Sexual abuse of wives. New York: Free Press, 1985.
33. Minnesota Department of Corrections. Task Force on Sexual Exploitation by Counselors and Therapists. Minnesota Legislative Report: 1985.
34. Burkhart BR, Stanton AL. Sexual aggression in acquaintance relationships. In: Russell G, ed. Violence in intimate relationships, Old Tappan, NJ: Spectrum Press, 1985.
35. Koss MP. The hidden rape victim: Personality, attitudinal and situational characteristics. Psych Women Quarterly 1985; 9:193–212.

36. Skogan WG. Issues in the measurement of victimization. Department of Justice, Bureau of Statistics. Pub. No. NCJ-74682. Washington, DC: US Govt. Printing Office, 1981.

37. Bureau of Justice Statistics. Criminal victimization in the United States, 1982. Publication No. NCJ-92820. Washington, DC: US Dept. of Justice, 1984.

38. Katz S, Mazur MA. Understanding the rape victim: A synthesis of research findings. New York: Wiley, 1979.

39. Bureau of Justice Statistics. The crime of rape. Washington, DC: US Dept. of Justice, 1985.

40. Law Enforcement Assistance Administration. Criminal victimization surveys in eight American cities. (Pub. No. SD-NCS-C5). Washington, DC: US Govt. Printing Office, 1975.

41. Russell DEH. Sexual exploitation: Rape, child sexual abuse, and work place harrassment. Beverly Hills, CA: Sage, 1984.

42. Koss MP, Gidycz CA, Wisniewski N. The scope of rape: Incidence and prevalence of sexual aggression and victimization in a national sample of higher education students. J Consulting Clin Psychology 1987; 55:162–170.

43. McDermott MJ. Rape victimization in 26 American cities. (Analytic Report SD-VAD-6) Department of Justice, Law Enforcement Assistance Administration. Washington, DC: US Govt. Printing Office, 1979.

44. Sparks RF. Research on victims of crime: Accomplishments, issues, and new directions. DHHS Publication No. (ADM) 82-1091. Washington, DC: US Govt. Printing Office, 1982.

45. Block CR, Block RL. Crime definition, crime measurement, and victim surveys. J Social Issues 1984; 40(1):137–159.

46. Garofalo J, Hindelang MJ. An introduction to the National Crime Survey. Washington, DC: National Criminal Justice Information and Statistics Service, Law Enforcement Administration, US Dept. of Justice, 1979, SD-VAD-4.

47. Catlin G, Murray S. Report on Canadian victimization survey methodological pretests. Ottawa: Statistics Canada, 1979.

48. Sparks RF, Glenn HG, Dodd DJ. Surveying victims. New York: Wiley, 1977.

49. Turner AG. The San Jose methods test of known crime victims. Washington, DC: National Criminal Justice Information and Statistics Service, Law Enforcement Assistance Administration, US Dept. of Justice, 1972.

50. Kilpatrick DG, Veronen LJ. Assessing victims of rape: Methodological issues. Final report, NIMH Grant No. 1 R01 MH38052. Rockville, MD: National Institute for Mental Health, 1984.

51. Ennis PH. Criminal victimization in the United States: A report of a national survey. The President's Commission on Law Enforcement and Administration of Justice, Field Surveys II. Washington, DC: US Govt. Printing Office, 1967.

52. Gottfredson MR, Hildelang MJ. A consideration of memory decay and telescoping biases in victimization surveys. J Criminal Justice 1977; 5:202–216.

53. Paez A. Criminal victimization in the United States. Washington, DC: Technical Report, Bureau of Justice Statistics, US Dept. of Justice, 1983.

54. Sudman S, Bradburn NM. Response effects in surveys: A review and synthesis. Chicago: Aldine, 1974.

55. Russell DEH. The prevalence and incidence of forcible rape and attempted rape of females. Victimology 1982; 7:81–93.

56. Ageton SC. Sexual assault among adolescents. Lexington, MA: Lexington Books, 1983.

57. Russell DEH. Incidence and prevalence of intrafamilial and extrafamilial sexual abuse of female children. Child Abuse Neglect 1983; 7:133–146.
58. Rada RT. Clinical aspects of the rapist. New York: Grune & Stratton, 1978.
59. Perdue WC, Lester D. Personality characteristics of rapists. Perceptual and Motor Skills 1972; 35:514.
60. Rader CM. MMPI profile types of exposers, rapists and assaulters in a court services population. J Consulting Clin Psychology 1977; 45:61–69.
61. Clark L, Lewis D. Rape: The price of coercive sexuality. Toronto: Women's Press, 1977.
62. Scully D, Marolla J. "Riding the bull at Gilley's": Convicted rapists describe the rewards of rape. Social Problems 1985; 32(3):251–263.
63. Malamuth NM, Donnerstein E, eds. Pornography and sexual aggression. Orlando, FL: Academic Press, 1984.
64. Koss MP, Leonard KE, Beezley DA, Oros CJ. Nonstranger sexual aggression: A discriminant analysis of the psychological characteristics of undetected offenders. Sex Roles 1985; 12:981–992.
65. Rapaport K, Burkhart BR. Personality and attitudinal characteristics of sexually coercive college males. J Abnormal Psychology 1984; 93:216–221.
66. Barlow DH. The treatment of sexual deviation: Toward a comprehensive behavioral approach. In: Calhoun KS, Adams HE, Mitchell KM, eds. Innovative treatment methods in psychopathology. New York: Wiley, 1974.
67. Brownell KD, Barlow DH. Behavioral treatment of sexual deviation. In: Foa E, Goldstein A, eds. Handbook of behavior modification. New York: Wiley, 1980.
68. Hayes S, Brownell K, Barlow D. Heterosocial skills training and covert sensitization: Effects on social skills and sexual arousal in sexual deviants. Behavior Res Ther 1983; 21:383–392.
69. Segal ZV, Marshall WL. Heterosexual social skills in a population of rapists and child molesters. J Consulting Clin Psychology 1985; 53:55–63.
70. Overholser JC, Beck S. Multi-method assessment of rapists, child molesters, and three control groups in behavioral and psychological measures. J Consulting Clin Psychology 1986; 54:682–687.
71. Malamuth NM. Predictors of naturalistic sexual aggression. J Personality Social Psychology 1986; 50:953–962.
72. Koss MP, Dinero TE. Predictors of sexual aggression among a national sample of male college students. Paper presented at the New York Academy of Sciences Conference, Human Sexual Aggression: Current Perspectives, New York City, 1987.
73. Finklehor D. Child sexual abuse: New theory and research. New York: Free Press, 1985.
74. Glaser D. Crime in our changing society. New York: Holt, Rinehart and Winston, 1979.
75. Deming MP, Eppy A. The sociology of rape. Sociology Social Res 1981; 65:357–380.
76. Amir M. Patterns in forcible rape. Chicago: University of Chicago Press, 1971.
77. Kanin EJ. Male aggression in dating-courtship relations. Am J Sociology 1957; 63:197–204.
78. Selkin J. Protecting personal space: Victim and resister reactions to assaultive rape. J Community Psychology 1978; 6:263–268.
79. Koss MP, Harvey M. The rape victim: Clinical and community approaches to treatment. Lexington, Massachusetts: Stephen Greene Press, 1987.

80. Feild HS. Attitudes toward rape: A comparative analysis of police, rapists, crisis counselors, and citizens. J Personality Social Psychology 1978; 36:156–179.

81. Scully D, Marolla J. Convicted rapists' vocabulary of motive: Excuse and justification. Social Problems 1984; 31:530–544.

82. Bart PB. A study of women who were raped and avoided rape. J Social Issues 1981; 37:123–137.

83. Weis K, Borges SS. Victimology and rape: The case of the legitimate victim. Issues in Criminology 1973; 8:72.

84. Reynolds JM. Rape as social control. Catalyst 1975; 8:62–67.

85. Malamuth NM. Rape proclivity among males. J Social Issues 1981; 37:138–157.

86. Sutherland S, Scherl D. Patterns of response among rape victims. Am J Orthopsychiatry 1970; 40:503–511.

87. Burgess AW, Holmstrom LL. Rape trauma syndrome. Am J Psychiatry 1974; 131:981–986.

88. Calhoun KS, Atkeson BM, Resick PA. A longitudinal examination of fear reactions in victims of rape. J Counseling Psychology 1982; 29:655–661.

89. Kilpatrick DG, Resick PA, Veronen LJ. Effects of a rape experience: A longitudinal study. J Social Issues 1981; 37(4):105–122.

90. Atkeson BM, Calhoun KS, Resick PA, Ellis EM. Victims of rape: Repeated assessment of depressive symptoms. J Consulting Clin Psychology 1982; 50:96–102.

91. Frank E, Turner SM, Duffy B. Depressive symptoms in rape victims. J Affective Disorders 1979; 1:269–297.

92. Becker JV, Abel GG, Skinner LJ. The impact of a sexual assault on the victim's sexual life. Victimology 1979; 4:229–235.

93. Becker JV, Skinner LJ. Assessment and treatment of rape-related sexual dysfunctions. Clinical Psychologist 1983; 36:102–105.

94. Feldman-Summers S, Gordon PE, Meagher JR. The impact of rape on sexual satisfaction. J Abnormal Psychology 1979; 88(1):101–105.

95. Resick PA, Calhoun KS, Atkeson B, Ellis EM. Social adjustment in victims of sexual assault. J Consulting Clin Psychology 1981; 49:705–712.

96. Nadelson CC, Notman MI, Zackson H, Gornick J. A follow-up study of rape victims. Am J Psychiatry 1982; 139:1266–1270.

97. Ellis EM, Atkeson BM, Calhoun KS. An assessment of long-term reaction to rape. J Abnormal Psychology 1981; 90:263–266.

98. American Psychiatric Association. Diagnostic and statistical manual of mental disorders (3rd ed., rev). Washington, DC: American Psychiatric Association, 1987.

99. Janoff-Bulman R. Characterological versus behavioral self-blame: Inquiries into depression and rape. J Personality Social Psychology 1979; 37:1798–1809.

100. Seigel JM, Burnam MA, Stein JA, Golding JM, Sorenson SB. Sexual assault and psychiatric disorders: A preliminary investigation. Final report for National Institute of Mental Health Grant, 1986.

101. George LK, Winfield-Laird J. Sexual assault: Prevalence and mental health consequences. Final Report submitted to National Institute of Mental Health, 1986.

102. Burgess AW, Holmstrom LL. Rape trauma syndrome. Am J Psychiatry 1974; 131:981–986.

103. Largen MA. The anti-rape movement: Past and present. In: Burgess AW, ed. Rape and sexual assault. New York: Garland, 1985.
104. Kilpatrick DG, Veronen LJ, Resick PA. Psychological sequelae to rape: Assessment and treatment strategies. In: Doleys DM, Meredith RL, Ciminero AR, eds. Behavioral medicine: Assessment and treatment strategies. New York: Plenum, 1982:473–497.
105. Frank E, Stewart BD. Treating depression in victims of rape. Clinical Psychologist 1983; 36:95–98.
106. Ochberg FM, ed. Post-traumatic therapy and victims of violence. New York: Brunner/Mazel, 1988.
107. Burgess AW, Holmstrom LL. Rape: Crisis and recovery. West Newton, MA: Awab, Inc., 1986.
108. Foley T. Family response to rape and sexual assault. In: Burgess AW, ed. Rape and sexual assault. New York: Garland, 1985.
109. Barlow DH, Wolfe BE. Behavioral approaches to anxiety disorders: A report on the NIMH-SUNY-Albany Research Conference. J Consulting Clin Psychology 1981; 49:448–454.
110. Swift CF. The prevention of rape. In: Burgess A, ed. Rape and sexual assault. New York: Garland, 1985.
111. Sanday PR. The socio-cultural context of rape: A cross-cultural study. J Social Issues 1981; 37:25.
112. Swift C. Sexual victimization of children: An urban mental health center survey. Victimology 1979; 2(2):322–327.
113. Groth AN. Men who rape. New York: Plenum, 1979.
114. Ressler R. Violent crime. FBI Law Enforcement Bulletin 1985; 54(8).
115. Seghorn T, Boucher RJ, Prentky RA. Childhood sexual abuse in the lives of sexually aggressive offenders. J Am Academy Child and Adolescent Psychiatry 1987; 26:262–267.
116. Horowitz MJ, ed. Stress response syndromes. New York: Jason Aronson, 1975.
117. Van der Kolk B, Boyd H, Krystal J, Greenberg M. Post-traumatic stress disorder as a biological based disorder: Implications of the animal model in inescapable shock. In: Van der Kolk B, ed. Post-traumatic stress disorder: Psychological and biological sequelae. Washington, DC: American Psychiatric Association Press, 1984.

6

Spouse Abuse

EVAN STARK AND ANNE H. FLITCRAFT

Spouse abuse (or interspousal violence) is defined as the use of physical force in intimate relationships among adults. Battering is defined as a syndrome of control and increasing entrapment attendant upon spouse abuse and characterized by a history of injury, general medical complaints, isolation, stress-related psychosocial problems, and unsuccessful help-seeking. Among the most commonly reported psychosocial problems linked to battering are rape, substance abuse, attempted suicide, depression, and child abuse. Either partner or both may be abused. To date, however, the syndrome of entrapment associated with battering has been identified as a problem only among women.

In measuring "spouse abuse," researchers disagree about whether to restrict themselves to intact or married couples and about which instances of force constitute "abuse." Whereas these differences shape society's response to domestic violence, in clinical settings battering should be suspected in any case in which the history or presenting problem indicates at least one instance of assault by any social partner regardless of sex, marital status, or living arrangements. Women are injured by abuse approximately 13 times as frequently as men. We retain the term "spouse," however, to indicate equal concern for men assaulted in intimate relations.

There are no periodic, standardized databases from which to reliably estimate the extent of spouse abuse. Estimates of its prevalence are based on a representative national survey and follow-up and on surveys of state and local populations. These sources offer widely discrepant estimates of how many men are abused, but consistently indicate that approximately 20 percent of adult women in the United States—perhaps as many as 15 million women—have been physically abused at least once by a male intimate.

Procedures to identify abuse are only very slowly being introduced in clinical settings. For this reason, epidemiological data based on diagnoses of abuse recorded in medical charts seriously underestimate the problem. One effective way to measure battering in clinical settings is by abstracting the adult trauma history from the medical records of a female patient population. Frank questioning supported by a full trauma history and by sensitivity to the signs of abuse also makes it possible to identify cases of battering in emergency and primary care sites.

Three models have developed to explain abuse. The interpersonal violence model emphasizes psychological deficits, psychosocial problems (such as alcoholism), and distorted interpersonal communication as causal factors, often linking these to current stressors (such as unemployment) or inherited behavior patterns. Psychotherapy is the preferred response. According to the family violence model, the intimacy and privacy that distinguish the family from other groups lead to high rates of "domestic violence," including spouse abuse. In this view, the root cause is normative support for physical punishment in childhood and for violence to resolve marital disputes. A combination of public education and tighter police controls over family behavior is called for. According to the gender-politics model, "violence against women" reflects an attempt by men—supported by discriminatory institutions—to maintain their already greater authority and privilege. This approach favors emergency shelter, the criminal prosecution of abusers, "empowerment," and giving survivors the resources and support needed to escape violence.

Clinical data indicate that abuse may be the single most important source of injury among women; that abuse is rarely an isolated episode; that abusive injury may be distinguished by its sexual nature rather than its severity; and that a range of psychosocial problems related to frustrated help-seeking and the stress of living in a violent home are frequent sequelae of abusive injury among women. Battering develops through stages characterized by increasing levels of danger, fear, isolation, and entrapment. The prevalence of abuse in virtually all clinical populations of women makes it a major context for rape, female alcohol and drug abuse, attempted suicide, child abuse, and mental illness.

Of the four components of prevention—shelter, law enforcement, legislation, and health care—the health response remains the least developed. There are potential roles for state and federal governments in broadening police and judicial power in abuse cases, funding shelters, educating the public about abuse, reducing inequities based on gender, and mandating training for health, law enforcement, and social service personnel.

The health response should begin by improving the identification and evaluation of abuse and by referring victims to appropriate services. Emphasis should shift from crisis intervention to primary care. Victim-blaming explanations and strategies should be eliminated. To prevent spouse abuse, however, the health sector must go beyond the traditional medical model of prevention to "complex social prevention." This entails joining with other institutional providers, including battered women's shelters, to modify such nonmedical factors as the use of firearms and gender biases in the law.

STATEMENT OF THE PROBLEM

The purposes of this chapter are to assess the distribution, impact, and dimensions of spouse abuse in various populations; to describe case identification; to evaluate the major causal explanations; and to sketch a strategy for prevention that includes a central role for health care. The clinical components and sequelae of abuse are also described, and antecedent problems or risk factors are evaluated for possible use in identifying and managing the problem.

Spouse abuse presents a challenge to epidemiology because its parameters are not well defined, its severity is highly subjective, its causes are poorly understood, and its psychosocial consequences are often linked in very complex ways to physical events. This helps explain why a problem that may affect as much as 20 percent of the adult female population and that results in more than three times as many injuries as auto accidents has been largely neglected by health researchers, including those specializing in injury.

Case identification requires that we specify which acts of force or violence constitute "abuse" and which relationships should be considered "spousal." The broadest definition of abuse is presented by Straus et al. (1). The Conflict Tactics Scale (CTS) they use to measure domestic violence includes any act of force, from threats and sibling fights through homicide. Berk et al. (2) criticize the CTS for failing to differentiate violent acts according to their intent or physical consequences and suggest that abuse be restricted to acts with a high probability of causing injury. At the other extreme, the National Crime Survey (NCS) asks only about acts that victims consider criminal assault. Finally, Stark et al. (3,4) argue that abuse should be considered whenever there is a complaint related to violence or control, regardless of whether injury is involved.

Differences are equally sharp about which assailant-victim relationships should be considered. For Straus et al. (1), the unique character of the family system merits an exclusive focus on intact couples. Feminists take a more catholic view, considering any relationship premised on inequalities in power as potentially abusive, including gay and dating relationships. Feminists also believe that, because social institutions support male authority, the peculiar process of entrapment reflected in battering affects women almost exclusively.

These differences have enormous consequences for our understanding and response to spouse abuse. Equating abuse with the broadest range of aggressive acts results in equivalent rates of victimization for women and men (1,5). By contrast, women appear to be victimized 13 times more frequently than men when only acts resulting in injury are considered (2), or when abuse is limited to episodes that men and women consider assaultive, i.e., the NCS criterion (6). Whereas individual or family-oriented interventions are favored by those who identify abuse with the family system, feminists, who consider family therapy ill-advised in cases of abuse, insist that responsibility for abuse be clearly identified, that abusers be punished, and that victims be protected and "empowered."

Definitions

Domestic violence is the category of acts under which spouse abuse and woman battering are normally classified. Definitions of violence differ with the context. Legal definitions include acts intended to cause physical pain or injury (assaults), threats (Connecticut Domestic Violence Response Act), acts against property (Seattle's Municipal Code), or the unjust usurpation of power. Less bound by community mores, research definitions may extend to any act of force (conflict tactics) and even to mental abuse (7). In clinical settings, an effective operational definition of violence or spouse abuse must rely on an inclusive notion of violence by an adult regardless of the severity of injury inflicted or whether it involves injury, psychosocial problems, or simply fear.

Legal differences about which relations are "domestic" focus on the age of cohabitants (Connecticut Domestic Violence Response Act) and on the fact, status, and length of cohabitation and range from present cohabitants only (Municipal Code, Richmond, Virginia) through all persons who are "social partners," defined by those who have a dating relationship whether or not they have cohabitated or have a child in common (Seattle's Municipal Code). For clinicians the central concern is future health risks, and the important differentiation is between an anonymous assault, mugging, or other street crime where further assault by the criminal is unlikely; and assault by any social partner regardless of sex, age, marital status, or cohabitation. In summary, although legal definitions may be more restrictive, a clinical definition of spouse abuse would include any act of force (including threats) for which social partners seek help.

Prefacing abuse with the generic term "spouse" indicates concern for males as well as females and for situations in which both partners are equally abusive (interspousal violence). Though far less frequently reported than wife abuse, husband abuse is a reality to which clinicians must be sensitive. Equally important is violence among gays or adolescent dating partners.

Battering refers to the etiology of a range of health problems that follow an initial episode of abuse. Stark (8) and Stark and Flitcraft (3,4,9,10) identify a battering syndrome among abused women. From a medical standpoint, the syndrome is established by an initial assault (abuse) followed by a history of injury, often including sexual assault, general medical complaints, psychological problems, and persistent help-seeking. Women who are separated, divorced, or single are at the highest risk of battering. No process comparable to battering has been observed among abused men. This suggests that woman abuse (which leads to battering) is clinically distinct from interspousal violence (mutual combat), husband abuse, and the range of tactics couples use to resolve conflicts.

Woman abuse is a problem with an extremely low spontaneous cure rate.

A Texas survey (11) found that only 25 percent of abused women escaped after a single episode of violence, and Stark et al. (3) report that 85 percent of the women in their medical case load who have ever been abused remain at risk. Still, 63 percent of the battered women in the Texas survey eventually escaped, a finding confirmed by Cambell (12).

In addition to being accompanied by a history of adult trauma, battering may present through chronic (and frustrated) help-seeking; nonspecific complaints of pain; injury during pregnancy; fear or anxiety associated with family conflict; isolation; and multiple psychosocial problems related to the stress of living in a violent home, including substance abuse, rape, child abuse, attempted suicide, and mental illness. The disproportionate risk of these problems among battered women appears primarily after the onset of abuse (4,8,13), which suggests that battering is the cause.

Why woman abuse leads so frequently to battering is unclear. Factors frequently mentioned include the inadequacy of current protections against violence, the survivor's fear of being killed if she leaves, the fear that children will be scapegoated, the lack of economic opportunity, the inappropriate and punitive responses of helping institutions, and the total control many batterers exercise over the material, sexual, and social lives of their victims (9).

DATA SOURCES

An important function of reliable prevalence data on spouse abuse is to determine unmet health and service needs. Although New York, New Jersey, and Connecticut have programs to train health care personnel to identify abuse, as yet there are no preexisting databases from which to derive reliable estimates of spouse abuse or woman battering. No widely recognized identification procedures have been adopted; and reporting is sporadic, even in states like Connecticut where it is mandated. Woman battering may be associated with the psychiatric diagnosis of posttraumatic stress disorder, (DSM IIIR) or battered adult syndrome, ICD code 995.81, but these diagnoses are rarely used. Another obstacle to developing uniform identification procedures and assessing unmet health needs is the aforementioned disagreement about how the problem should be defined and measured. One issue, for example, is whether to expend resources in clinical settings to identify husband abuse (which has been documented by surveys), although there are no survey data indicating that men view husband abuse as a serious problem.

Estimates of the most severe forms of spousal violence—homicide and assault—can be gleaned from the Federal Bureau of Investigation's (FBI) Uniform Crime Reports (UCR) and the National Crime Survey (NCS) taken each year by the Department of Justice. The UCR is particularly helpful in identifying aggravated assault and homicide. However, UCR data do not indicate whether or not the victim and perpetrator live together—a common criterion in distinguishing domestic violence—and only include problems reported to the police and the FBI, a small proportion of all spousal assault. By contrast, the NCS, a general population survey, records many crimes not reported to the police and includes data on medical treatment, characteristics of the victim-offender relationship, and whether or not police are notified. NCS estimates of spousal violence may be low (6), perhaps because respondents are often questioned in the presence of their spouses and because respondents may misinterpret the emphasis on "criminal" acts as excluding domestic violence. Still, the NCS is particularly useful in detecting what the use of force means to victims, e.g., whether they think an assault has occurred. From this vantage, it is significant that where the rates of severe violence against women detected by the NCS and Straus et al. (1) are identical (3.9% and 3.8%), the rate of husband abuse identified by the NCS is only 0.3%, a tiny fraction of the rate of husband abuse identified by Straus et al. (4.6%) when they asked about all aggressive acts. This suggests that whereas women consider men assaultive when they use force to resolve conflicts, men classify only a handful of episodes where women use force as assaultive, possibly because weapons are involved.

Although there are no periodic surveys of spousal violence, representative surveys provide useful estimates of interspousal violence, husband abuse, and wife abuse (1,14–17). State surveys are another reliable source on woman abuse (11,18,19). These surveys primarily provide information about instances of force (abuse), but they do not identify needs for service or inform about whether and how often abuse evolves into a syndrome of control and entrapment (battering).

Hospital-based Data Sources

Gathering data on spouse abuse in health care settings for the purpose of case identification is important both clinically and epidemiologically. For those involved directly in service delivery, case identification and data collection methods begin with the patient encounter but may extend to a complete review of the patient's medical records to understand the history and extent of abuse and to document the patient's previous attempts to find aid. Thus far, no attempts have been made to use medical records to identify intraspousal violence or husband abuse. However, medical record reviews have been used to estimate the number of abused women using the service of a particular clinic or medical center, how many are being recognized, and the major medical and mental health problems of this population. The record review can also document the current response in a given medical or mental health complex to both recognized and unrecognized victims of domestic assault.

Epidemiological Research in Health Care Settings

Accurate epidemiological data on domestic assault are difficult to gather in clinical settings. Since physicians rarely record abuse or list it as a diagnosis in medical records, incidence data based on physician reporting or discharge diagnoses seriously and consistently underestimate the magnitude of the problem. A critical review of medical records, however, permits the trained researcher to identify both abused women and women whose medical histories are suggestive of domestic violence. Where there is access to a consolidated medical records system that lists all visits, including those to the emergency service, the potential battered women or women at risk for battering may be identified by a retrospective review of the full medical records of a sample of adult women. In this review women should be defined as at risk for abuse if their history contains at least one episode attributed to an assault by a male intimate or family member ("positives"); an assaultive episode not attributed to street crime ("probables"); or a recorded alleged etiology that is inconsistent with the injury presentation ("suggestives"). First developed at Yale New Haven Hospital (20), this method has been used with consistent results at Waterbury Hospital (21), the Medical College of Pennsylvania (22,23), and the Philadelphia Health Management Corporation (24).

Case Identification in Health Care Settings

Early claims that abused women delay or fail to report injuries have not been sustained. Indeed, abusive injury is reported more promptly than injuries from auto accidents (8). Sensitive probing can evoke an accurate patient account of abuse as a source of injury. After staff training and the introduction of an identification protocol in the emergency department at the Medical College of Pennsylvania, the percentage of women found to be battered increased almost sixfold, from 5.6 percent to 30 percent (23).

In screening abused women, frank questioning to elicit a history of deliberate assault (frequently associated with previous episodes of trauma) is the most important step in patient identification. The routine use of a trauma history avoids the problem of identifying abuse only after the extent and nature of the injuries make the diagnosis obvious—situations representing only the severest injuries.

In addition, since the majority of health visits by abused women are to nonemergency primary care sites, a protocol that outlines identification procedures and delineates responsibilities for assessment and referral should be introduced at all primary care and general medical and mental health clinics as well as at emergency medical and psychiatric settings.

Battering should be part of the differential diagnosis of every encounter with an injured client. The direct questions "Has someone done this to you?" and "Have you been injured before?" are appropriate in all cases of injury. Some specific aspects of the presentation should heighten the clinician's "index of suspicion" and prompt frank discussion with the client regarding possible problems with domestic assault. These include multiple injuries, central injuries (head, neck, breast, chest, abdomen, perineum), rape, and the presentation of medically insignificant trauma or injury during pregnancy. The hallmark of abuse is the sexual nature of the injuries inflicted, not their severity.

Another clue to abuse is a patient's accumulation of quasi-medical labels such as "hysterical," "crock," "hypochondriac," or "patient with vague complaints." In the medical emergency service, complaints indicating abuse may be associated with "old" injuries, particularly to the back, neck, or ribs; diffuse trauma that does not leave anatomical evidence but results in complaints of headache or nonspecific pain; sleep disorders, anxiety, dysphagia, hyperventilation, or other problems symptomatic of the stress associated with living in a violent environment; and alcohol or drug abuse.

In medical clinics where records are kept more consistently than in emergency settings, clues to abuse include persistent visits with vague complaints, frequent use of minor tranquilizers and sleep medication, increasing reliance upon alcohol, or abuse of licit or illicit drugs. In obstetrical and gynecology clinics, a history that should prompt the clinician's suspicion of abuse includes self-induced or attempted abortions, multiple therapeutic abortions, miscarriages, and divorce or separation during pregnancy. Persistent gynecological complaints, particularly abdominal pain and dyspareunia in the context of normal physical and laboratory exams, are frequently overlooked manifestations of domestic violence. It is the clustering and repetition of presentations and complaints rather than isolated events that are significant. Although using medical records as we have outlined is a laborious process, it can prove invaluable to health personnel in both the day-to-day treatment of battered women and in the development of a prevention-oriented protocol and service.

CAUSES AND RISK FACTORS

Explanatory Models

The literature on domestic violence is characterized by a wealth of descriptive material and a dearth of systematic theorizing (or theory testing) (cf. 3,13,25–28). Three explanatory models emerge from attempts to summarize this vast body of material (9,29–32).

Interpersonal Violence Model

According to the interpersonal violence model, violence arises among adults who lack the skills to cope appropriately and nonviolently with stress or conflict. Personal, psychological, and family deficits, either alone or in combination, make certain individuals (or families) "violence prone" in response to events perceived as personal or family crises, such as unemployment or the birth of a child. Assailants and victims are distinguished by behavioral problems such as depression and substance abuse, a history of violence, neglect, or sexual abuse in childhood, and/or a personality profile that includes immaturity, hostility, an inability to communicate, lack of empathy, and low self-esteem. Since this model assumes that violence (or the need to control) has underlying behavioral or psychiatric causes, interventions are focused on these causes of violence, rather than on violence per se. Individual, couples, or family systems therapy; cognitive-behavioral work with batterers or alcoholics; and programs designed to teach mothers of abused children how to parent more effectively illustrate this approach.

Three related empirical propositions follow from this theory, that victims and assailants suffer psychological and/or behavioral problems disproportionately, that these problems provide the context for abuse (and not the reverse), and that batterers and their victims have a distinctive personality profile, family history, or pattern of relating.

That battered women suffer disproportionate rates of various problems is well established. Stark et al. (4) found that, compared to nonbattered women, battered women in the medical population have a disproportionate risk of alcohol abuse (15% vs. 1%), drug abuse (9% vs. 1%), attempted suicide (12% vs. 1%), various mental health problems, and experience with abuse in childhood (15% vs. 1%). Moreover, the self-blame and impaired self-esteem that are hallmarks of other posttraumatic stress disorders appear to characterize at least those abused women who use mental health services (33). There is also evidence that a disproportionate number of those who experience violence as children either become abusive or are abused as adults (1,34).

However, many writers attribute a causal role to this "pathology" without determining whether the pathology precedes the onset of abuse (35) or how significant a percentage of victims or assailants even evidence the problem in question. In fact, battered women evidence a disproportionate risk of serious psychosocial problems only after the onset of abuse (8,9), and neither the majority of batterers nor their victims evidence a distinctive or multi-problem profile either as children or during the abusive relationship (9,36). Many populations of abuse victims do not evidence self-blame or low self-esteem, and some evidence suggests that self-blame may be a coping mechanism associated with positive psychological outcomes for survivors of abuse (37-40), a way of taking control where control is severely limited (41). At most, then, psychopathology is the context for violence in only a small percentage of instances.

Family Violence Model

The family violence model, identified primarily with the pioneering work of sociologists Murray Straus, Richard Gelles, and Suzanne Steinmetz, contends that intrafamilial violence is distinctive because of the unique nature of the family as an institution, particularly its emphasis on intimacy and privacy, and because it is more frequent, intense, and all-encompassing than violence in other settings. This theory suggests that normative support for violence as a means to settle disputes combines with the choice of the family as a setting to resolve problems about which people feel deeply until all family members, including siblings, become enmeshed in a violent pattern. Violence is learned in childhood, transmitted across generations, reinforced by a host of cultural institutions, and provoked by current stressors such as poverty or unemployment. The theory also acknowledges that men generally inflict greater physical harm than other family members. Because family members tend to conceal their violence due to fear and a belief in privacy, risk factors must be identified and monitored.

This approach finds support in survey data implicating women as well as men in homicides and assaults and in evidence that women seek help for as few as one in five assaults (18). The very different meaning, consequences, and dynamics of wife abuse, husband abuse, child abuse, elder abuse, and sibling fights are less important than their common denominator—the use of force as a tactic in conflicts among cohabitants. Survey data indicate a prevalence of such acts ranging from 4 percent for abuse of the elderly to 80 percent for sibling violence. Moreover, disproportionate numbers of both batterers and their victims were abused as children. And violence is disproportionately linked to such common indicators of stress as low income, minority status, status inconsistency, and substance abuse.

But the major claims of this model have not been supported. No connection has been shown, for example, between survey data on acts of force by various family members and any single set of outcomes, including injuries and requests for health and other services. Elder abuse is primarily a problem of institutional care, not family life (9), and the majority of child abusers are the same men who are beating the child's mother, which again points away from family dynamics as such (9). Even more important, whereas women apparently use force as a conflict tactic as frequently as men, they report being assaulted by their spouse 13 times more frequently (6), suggesting that men and women attach very different meanings to acts of force. The vast majority of abused children do not become violent adults (or victims) (42), and the vast majority of adults currently involved in violence were not abused or neglected as children (34). Finally, advocates of this model have cited delay or failure to report as more evidence of the pathological status of battered women. However, evidence from medical records indicates that victims report woman abuse promptly (4), and that the infrequent mention of abuse on official records is explained more readily by institutional neglect than by a failure to report (24).

The Gender-Politics Model

An unresolved question is whether the family is unique as a setting for violence or whether violence that occurs within families is just one instance of a more widespread phenomenon. The gender-politics model contends that violence in the family is merely a special instance of a pattern of male control (over women, children, or even other men) that extends from dating relationships through parenting and marriage to economic life. Violence is an option some men choose when they feel their privileged access to scarce resources (like money or sex) threatened by female independence or when women fail to fulfill perceived domestic responsibilities. Women may fight back or even initiate violence. However, because woman abuse occurs in the context of unequal power and is supported by other discriminatory practices, its distinctive consequences include entrapment and the myriad psychosocial problems associated with the stress, anger, and fear of living with violence. Women stay in abusive relationships less because of their psychopathology and more because fear, lack of support, victim-blaming interventions, and the absence of resources combine to make mere survival more practical than escape. To challenge male authority in relationships as well as in other social arenas requires tough political choices—identification and punishment of male violence, support for the community-based shelter movement, and female empowerment.

Support for the gender-politics theory is compelling. Clinical data implicate male violence and control rather than a peculiar subset of violent families in the most significant health problems associated with abuse. Perhaps a million women turn to health care annually simply because of the physical effects of abuse (4,8), a figure many times greater than comparable figures for abused males, the elderly, or even abused children. Nor does the psychosocial syndrome of battering found among abused women appear to have a clinical counterpart among other groups, suggesting that only women become entrapped.

Gender relations rather than family dynamics are implicated by two further facts: single, divorced, and separated women are actually at a greater risk of abuse than married women (8,9), and women are injured as frequently by dating violence as by marital violence (43). Evidence that men may also be the major perpetrators of child abuse as well as of elder abuse suggests that these problems may also be rooted in male control (34,44). The thesis that many men perceive female status or independence as threatening is supported by the greater risk of violence to women whose education or income is higher than their partner's (status inconsistency) and by the frequency with which fights in violent homes concern "Who's boss?" (45).

Demographic Dimensions

Race

Black women are more likely to be abused than white women. Population surveys suggest that battering is two to three times as common among blacks as among whites (1,18), and a higher proportion of blacks than whites seek medical help because of battering as well (8). Black women, however, are also twice as likely to report their problem (18). It is unclear whether this excess risk is a function of race, income, or other factors. Among groups with similar income, blacks were actually less likely than whites to experience spousal violence (46).

Income, Occupation, and Status

Studies consistently show an inverse, but relatively small, relation between income and domestic violence. Certain white collar occupations (or occupational environments) may be associated with elevated risk, and status inconsistency—or a relationship in which the woman has a job higher in status than the man's job—may increase a woman's chance of being victimized.

Risk Factors

Most research on domestic violence fails to establish the clear temporal sequence necessary to show that a characteristic such as low self-esteem is a cause or risk factor rather than an outcome of spouse abuse. For this reason, the following personality, demographic, and social factors are best understood as what Brown and Harris (47) term "vulnerability factors." Whereas such factors cannot produce domestic violence and may have no effect on it at all, they do appear to interact with the situational dynamics in domestic conflict, often in ways that are still poorly understood.

Personality Traits
Studies with the most reliable designs report few if any significant personality differences between battered and nonbattered women. No consistent personality profile has been identified for battered women. Where some turn anger inward, a substantial number are outwardly aggressive, independent, or overtly hostile to their assailants. Early psychiatric studies straightforwardly adopted the stereotyped view that battered women were masculine, frigid, overly emotional, with weakened ties to reality, or that they evidenced role reversal and inappropriate sexual expression (48). But in matched comparison studies, these findings have not been replicated (49,50). Indeed, several studies find that abuse victims have a better sense of reality than their assailants (45), that they are more social and sympathetic than controls (49), and that they exhibit greater ego strength (51). Although there is some evidence that abused women have low self-esteem, little support is found for the view that battered women blame themselves for violence (52,53). Neither has subsequent research (8,40,54) supported early claims that battered women exhibited a "helplessness syndrome" (7) characterized by delayed reporting (55).

Social Class
Despite early evidence that domestic violence is prevalent in upper- and middle-class communities, survey and client studies consistently report higher rates of abuse among poor, unemployed, or working class groups (1,56–58). However, the most exacting study of this relation finds only a 3 percent difference between spousal violence reported by low-income women (11%) and women with family incomes of $25,000 or above (8%), with 10 percent of middle income women reporting abuse (18). Although the national representative sample surveys by Straus et al. (1) showed that drinking, approval of violence, and blue collar status had a cumulative relation to violence with the highest rates appearing when all three were present, occupational class itself was not significantly related to wife abuse (28). Status inconsistency may also increase women's vulnerability, regardless of whether a woman's status is

higher or lower than the male's or whether it is internally inconsistent (e.g., if her education is high and job status is low) (59). Indeed, the highest rates of abuse have been found among professional men who feel "unappreciated" by their lower status wives. By contrast, batterers are no more likely than other men to have inconsistent status (15,59).

Age

Age is inversely related to acts of domestic violence. Although acts of domestic violence are more common among couples under age 30 than among 31- to 50-year-olds (1,60), age does not differentiate battered from nonbattered women in clinical populations (4,61). In a study of battered women in a Philadelphia emergency department, McLeer and Anwar (23) found that where 42 percent of the female trauma patients 18–20 years of age were battered, 18 percent of the women over 60 were as well. Teens and the elderly represent high-risk populations whose battering is often misidentified as child abuse or elder abuse.

Marital Status

Married women are the least likely, and single, separated, and divorced women the most likely, to experience assault by a male intimate. Early surveys assessed domestic violence only among intact couples, reinforcing the mistaken belief that wives were the primary targets of battering (1,18).

A Texas survey (11) indicated that 25 percent of the women abused during the previous year and 63 percent of those ever abused have divorced or permanently left their husbands or live-in partners. But without adequate protection, separation or divorce may actually increase a woman's risk. The NCS data (6) show that separated women are the most vulnerable to assault, with divorced women next and married women last. Among women seeking medical assistance, victims were separated, single, or divorced at the time of 73 percent of the abusive injuries. Conversely, whereas only 16 percent of all assaults among married women are domestic, 55 percent of assaults among separated women are by a male intimate.

Social Situation

Violent couples and battered women are consistently reported to be more isolated than controls (8,62), a particular problem among military families (63). Since isolation often results from ongoing abuse, however, this may not be a vulnerability factor.

Pregnancy

Pregnancy is a high-risk period among abused women. Although family pressures, including the number of children, are frequently cited risk factors for battering, battered women presenting in the medical complex average no more children than controls (8). They are, however, pregnant nearly twice as often, one possible consequence of sexual assault; significantly more likely to have had a miscarriage or an abortion; and more likely to be pregnant at the time of injury (4). Twenty-eight percent of the abused women in the Texas survey were beaten while pregnant (11).

Between 20 percent and 25 percent of all obstetrical patients are abused women (4,64,65), a higher percentage than in the emergency service.

Alcohol

Alcohol is typically the consequence rather than the context for victimization among women. For batterers, although excessive drinking is associated with higher rates of wife abuse, alcohol is not typically an immediate antecedent of violence. Cessation of alcohol use does not appear to affect abusive behavior.

The correlation of alcohol use and abusive behavior has been frequently demonstrated (50); research suggests that 25–68 percent of all batterers use alcohol (13,66), and reported violence rates among men who use alcohol are two to 15 times higher than rates among abstainers (67,68). Still, literature reviews by Byles (67) and Orne and Rimmer (69) conclude that a causal role for alcohol cannot be supported. Moreover, alcohol appears to be involved in only 6–8 percent of the family disputes in which police are involved (70,71). Although Kantor and Straus (28) found that alcohol was involved in about one in four instances of wife abuse and that "high" and "binge" drinkers had a two to three times higher rate of assaulting their wives, 80 percent of the men in both the high and binge groups did not hit their wives during the sample year. A causal role for alcohol should be reflected in the effect of alcohol treatment on violence. However, Richardson and Cambell (72) reported that neither length of sobriety nor membership in Alcoholics Anonymous (AA) were linked to any reduction in male violence. Indeed, long-term AA members are less likely than short-term members to attribute responsibility for abuse to the factor of intoxication (73).

Violence in the Family of Origin

Violence in the family of origin increases both a woman's vulnerability and a man's propensity to abuse his wife and/or children. But the vast majority of persons who experience violence as children are not involved in violent relationships, and the typical batterer was neither abused as a child nor came from a violent home.

There is a widespread belief that the majority of today's violent couples are those who were brought up by parents who were violent to each other, and further, that children who are abused grow up to be abusing parents (1). Survey and case-control studies report significant correlations between current victimization and a woman's abuse as a child (1,18,60). Stark and Flitcraft (34) compared the pediatric records of battered and nonbattered women and found that the abuse victims had an excess risk of childhood mistreatment fourteen times higher than expected (15% to 1%) and concluded that childhood abuse was both a sensitive and a specific indicator of woman's vulnerability to abuse. However, two well-designed studies using multiple comparison groups and collecting data from men and women found no significant effect of childhood violence on later victimization (50,74). Straus et al. (1) presented data from their national sample demonstrating that men from violent childhoods (5% of the population) are ten times more likely to abuse their wives than men from nonviolent childhoods. However, consideration of the relative size of violent and nonviolent groups (5% and 37%) reveals that a current batterer is more than twice as likely to have had a nonviolent as a violent childhood and seven times more likely to come from a nonviolent than a violent home. Indeed, even 80 percent of the children from families Straus et al. (1) classify as "most violent" do not become batterers. Kaufman and Zigler (42) are more conservative in estimating that 30 percent of those abused as children become violent toward their own children.

The Medical Response

Neglect, denial, mistreatment, and punitive interventions and referrals characterize the ongoing care of women who present with abusive injury, responses that increase a woman's risk and reinforce denial, minimization, abuse, and victim-blaming by the batterer. A failure to identify battered women in health and mental health settings has been documented from medical records (3), patient interviews (75-76), and/or observation of doctor-patient encounters (24). In Connecticut, for example, where hospitals are required to file monthly reports of abuse cases, Yale-New Haven Hospital reported 79 cases of abuse for the six months ending in January 1985, approximately one in 12 of the cases of battering uncovered in the same hospital by Stark et al. (3) from a medical record review. When Hilberman questioned patients at a rural clinic in North Carolina, she discovered that only one in 15 of the abused women had been previously identified (75). In addition, records reviews, patient interviews, and direct observation reveal that health providers are more likely to refer battered than nonbattered women to psychiatry, to apply either traditional female labels (such as "hysteric") or other denigrating stigmata ("crock"), to prescribe tranquilizers and pain medication (4), and to institutionalize them in state mental hospitals.

Battered mothers of abused children are more likely than nonbattered mothers to have their children placed in foster care (34), and battered women who attempt suicide are more likely to be sent home with no follow-up than nonbattered women (8). At advanced stages of battering, clinicians interpret the sequelae of abuse as its cause and may intervene to manage these secondary problems (such as alcoholism) in ways that actually aggravate a victim's predicament.

A profile of violent couples based on a combination of low income, minority status, unemployment, status inconsistency, alcoholism, and a family history of violence might prove to be a sensitive indicator of spouse abuse. But its lack of specificity prevents such a profile from aiding identification, particularly in police, medical, mental health, or other multi-problem caseloads. By contrast, a history of victimization by male violence (an episode of woman abuse) and a history of frustrating helping encounters are the best predictors of woman battering.

OUTCOMES

Survey Results

Spouse Abuse
Approximately 12–20 percent of all couples experience interspousal violence that might be classified as abuse. To date, only one representative United States survey has specifically measured violent acts among cohabitants. Sampling 3,520 families in 1975, Straus et al. (1) estimate that 3.9 million instances of spouse abuse occur annually, that 3.8 percent or 1.8 million wives are abused by husbands, and that 4.6 percent or 2.2 million husbands are abused. An estimated 12.6 percent have ever experienced a "severe" violent episode (six million couples), and 28 percent report some use of force. In a ten-year follow-up telephone sample of 6,000 couples, Gelles and Straus (77) reported that the incidence rate of wife beating has fallen, though the decline is not statistically significant, whereas the rate of husband abuse has remained the same.

Two other surveys present similar results. An estimated 20 percent of the adult residents of Suffolk County, Long Island, have hit or been hit by their spouse (78). Meanwhile, Szinovacz (15) found that 26 percent of the women but 30 percent of the men had been abused in a sample of 103 couples from Pennsylvania towns. However, in a random survey of couples in Delaware, Steinmetz (79) found no cases of husband abuse.

Woman Abuse
Between 20 percent and 25 percent of the adult women in the United States—more than 12 million women—are at risk of being abused by a male intimate. A Harris Poll of Kentucky housewives (18) found that 10 percent had been abused during the year (80,000 women) and 21 percent had been abused during their lifetime. A North Carolina survey reported an identical number of women abused by "a person they knew," and slightly higher percentages have been reported using varying definitions of abuse in Pennsylvania (26%) and Texas (29%) (11,15). The NCS (6) found that the annual rate of domestic assault was 3.9 percent, virtually identical to the findings of Straus et al. By contrast, the NCS figure for men who report being assaulted by their partner is 0.3 percent, 15 times less than the comparable figure from Straus et al. (1) on husband abuse (4.6%), and 13 times less than the NCS figure on woman abuse.

Frequency
There are no consistent findings on the frequency or severity of interspousal violence or husband abuse, but woman abuse is characterized by frequent

beatings, often requiring medical attention. Forty-seven percent of the husbands who beat their wives do so three or more times a year (1). Similarly, NCS data (80) and the Texas survey indicate that between 25 percent and 30 percent of all abused women suffer "serial victimization"; many are beaten as frequently as once a week. Although knives and guns are not typically used in abusive incidents, they often are (1). And sexual assault frequently accompanies physical abuse. According to a survey of ever-married women in San Francisco, 14 percent had been raped by their current or former husbands (81,82). Still, the physical trauma inflicted by abuse is often medically insignificant. The emergency lies in the context: in these relationships, physical assault punctuates a history of control that extends from sexuality through money, friendships, food and clothing, work, and access to children.

Dating Violence

Patterns of violence and injury among dating couples are comparable to patterns among cohabitants. Studies of violence among unmarried persons have focused on college students almost exclusively, terming reported abuse "premarital" or "courtship" violence. Among the many studies in this genre, two using random samples found that 19 percent and 31.5 percent respectively were victims of physical aggression (83,84), whereas Makepeace (43) reported that 46 percent of those experiencing a violent episode suffered injury, with 5 percent requiring medical care. In a sample of 393 couples about to be married, O'Leary (5) reported that 42 percent of the women and 33 percent of the men had engaged in at least one act of physical aggression toward their partner in the previous year, a rate that is considerably higher than rates reported by married individuals. Interestingly, the physically aggressive couples also reported relatively high marital satisfaction, suggesting that aggression (which may be a necessary aspect of negotiation) has a very different meaning to couples than assault or abuse (which implies a violation of trust).

The Medical Context

There are no clinical reports of abused or battered husbands in a medical context. Medical assessments have focused exclusively on woman battering or on the link between spouse abuse and child abuse.

Frequency and Severity

Battering may be the single most common cause of injury for which women seek medical attention, accounting for more injury episodes than auto accidents, muggings, and rape combined. Abusive injury is typically ongoing and is distinguished by its sexual nature, not its severity.

Stark and Flitcraft reviewed the complete medical records of 3,676 women randomly selected from among female patients presenting with injury at a major metropolitan emergency room during one year (4,8). Although a mere 1 percent (n = 73) of the 5,040 injury episodes ever presented by these women were identified by clinical staff as due to abuse, a review of the adult trauma history revealed that 40 percent of the injury episodes were either identified by victims as resulting from a deliberate assault by an intimate (50% of the episodes), or this could be surmised from the circumstances. The authors concluded that 19 percent of the women presenting at the service had a history of abuse. This percentage was compared to 11 percent presenting with injuries resulting from auto accidents, usually thought to be the most common source of serious injury. By contrast with the institutional prevalence of 19 percent, just 4 percent of the women presented during the year with their first at-risk episode, what might be termed the institutional incidence. In other words, 75–80 percent of the battering cases brought to medical attention are ongoing.

Using the same identification technique, 25.7 percent of the emergency trauma cases at the Medical College of Pennsylvania (23) and 17 percent of the women in four Philadelphia emergency departments were found to be at risk for abuse (85). Following the introduction of an identification protocol at the Medical College of Pennsylvania, 30 percent of the emergency trauma caseload were diagnosed as battered, one of the highest percentages reported in any patient population (23). These findings corroborate Appleton (86).

Battered women are 13 times more likely than nonbattered women to be injured in the breast, chest, and abdomen and three times as likely to be injured while pregnant, an injury pattern suggesting the sexual nature of domestic violence (4). Frequent medical visits—particularly with "vague complaints"—and an extended medical history are direct functions of ongoing abuse. Almost one battered woman in five has presented at least 11 times with trauma, and another 23 percent have brought six to ten abusive injuries to the attention of clinicians (8). Still, abusive injuries are no more likely to result in hospitalization than nonabusive injuries, suggesting that in itself severity is not a good indicator of abuse.

Medical Utilization

The greatest proportion of medical visits by battered women do not involve trauma but general medical, behavioral, and psychiatric presentations. Battered women were more likely to present with depression, anxiety, family/marital/sexual problems (19% vs. 8%), and "vague medical complaints" (12% vs. 3%) (4). As a result, nontrauma medicine provides most of their care. For example, 25 percent of all obstetrical patients are abused women, as high a percentage as in the emergency service (8). Clearly, spouse abuse protocols should not be limited to emergency or trauma settings.

Alcohol and Drug Abuse

Battered women experience a rate of alcoholism and drug abuse that is significantly greater than nonbattered women. As a result, battering appears to be the single most important context yet identified for female alcoholism, possibly associated with 50 percent of all female alcoholism.

The association of alcohol abuse among women with adverse life events has long been recognized, but without the connection to violence being observed. However, Hilberman and Munson (75) observed that women patients in a nearby alcohol rehabilitation program were nearly all victims of marital or parental violence. Even prior to the first abusive episode appearing on the medical record, the rate of alcoholism is significantly greater among battered than among nonbattered women (4% vs. 1%), suggesting that female alcohol use may contribute to the onset of violence in some cases. By contrast, after the onset of abuse, alcoholism is 16 times as common among battered women. Indeed, abused women who developed alcohol problems had a higher rate of emergency medical utilization than any other population (4). Although battered women evidence no more drug abuse than nonbattered women prior to the onset of abuse, their risk becomes nine times greater than expected once an abusive episode has been presented to the hospital (4). Gerson (87) estimates that in fully 43 percent of the incidents of alcohol-related spouse abuse, the female victim had been drinking, although Kantor and Straus (28) found that at the time of the most serious violent incident, women alone had been drinking in only 2 percent of the cases and both spouses were drinking in 8 percent. Extrapolating from their stratified random sample, Stark and Flitcraft (4) estimate that 40 percent to 50 percent of all female alcoholism seen in emergency medical and psychiatric services may be precipitated by abuse.

Unfortunately, "AOB" (alcohol on breath) is a frequent reason given by clinicians for dismissing a woman's abuse. In addition, once a battered woman develops an alcohol or drug problem, the violence is seen as the consequence of the substance abuse, often a mistaken presumption (24).

Suicide Attempts

Attempted suicide—and particularly multiple attempts—is a significant sequela of abuse among women, affecting one abused woman in ten. Conversely, abuse may be the single most important precipitant for female suicide attempts yet identified.

Descriptive studies of battered women report that between 35 percent and 40 percent attempt suicide (7,35,88). Though there are no differences with respect to suicide risk factors between battered and nonbattered women prior to the first reported episode of abuse, subsequently battered women experience a relative risk of attempted suicide that is 4.8 times as high. Of the 10 percent who attempted suicide, 50 percent did so more than once (4,8). Twenty-six percent of female suicide attempts presented at the hospital in a year are associated with battering, whereas 50 percent of the black women who attempt suicide are abused. The battered women (26% of the population) account for 42 percent of all traumatic attempts and are significantly more likely to attempt suicide more than once (20% vs. 8%). Eighty-five percent of these women are seen in the hospital for at least one abusive injury prior to their first suicide attempt, highlighting the importance of abuse as a precipitating factor as well as the importance of early identification of abuse in suicide prevention. Furthermore, 44 percent mention marital conflict as the precipitating factor and over 80 percent of those mentioning marital conflict have been physically abused (4,8).

Rape

Abuse is among the most important precipitants of rape. Descriptive studies frequently include sexual assault as a factor in abusive relationships (81). Although rape is a relatively rare event in medical settings, almost one-third of the rape victims seen in the hospital have a documented history of abuse, and among rape victims over 30 years of age, 58 percent are battered women (8,89).

Child Abuse

Woman battering may be the single most important source of child abuse. In these cases, the majority of assailants are male batterers.

The impact of battering on children includes a number of psychological and behavioral problems, including internalizing behavior, nervousness and sadness, anxiety disorders, depression, nightmares, respiratory distress, and a range of somatic complaints (75,90-92). However, there are sharply discrepant findings about the frequency of child abuse among battered women, possibly due to definitional differences. Straus et al. (1) reported that the risk of child abuse is 12 percent higher where the husband hits his wife; Stewart and deBlois (93) found child abuse was two times as common among battered women as among nonbattered women; and Stark and Flitcraft (34) reported that battered women were five times as likely as nonbattered women to mention "fear of child abuse" to their clinician. Estimates of the exact frequency also differ widely. Thus, whereas Levine (91) uncovered physical abuse among only 1.7 percent of the children of battered mothers in his private practice, Hilberman and Munson (75) found that fully a third of the children in a rural population had been physically or sexually abused, and Bowker et al. (94) found that 70 percent of the battered women in a volunteer sample (n = 725) reported that the batterer also abused the children.

Even if child abuse is relatively rare in battering relationships, the prevalence of adult battering makes battering a major source of child abuse. In a review of a year's sample of mothers whose children had been "darted" for suspected physical abuse or neglect (n = 116), Stark and Flitcraft (9,34) reported that 45 percent were battered women, the highest percentage of battered women identified in any client population.

Interestingly, although there are no papers in the child abuse literature targeting male child abusers (95) and child abuse programs target mothers almost exclusively, men probably comprise the majority of child abusers, particularly where the mother is battered. Comparing medical examiner records in child abuse cases for two time periods, 1971–1973 and 1981–1983, Bergman et al. (96) reported that the proportion of known male perpetrators had risen from 38 percent to 49 percent of all cases and from 30 percent to 64 percent in severe cases. Survey evidence indicates that men are the assailants in from 25 percent to 55 percent of all reported cases (44,97,98), a remarkable finding given women's responsibility for most child rearing. Stark and Flitcraft (9,34) found that physical abuse (as opposed to neglect) was more than twice as likely among the children of battered mothers, and that fathers or father substitutes were three times as likely to be the abusing parents in these families. Finally, Bowker et al. (94) reported a strong relationship between male dominance in the previous year and spousal child abuse. This finding provides support for the gender-politics thesis.

The Mental Health Context

Severe mental health problems and disproportionate utilization of emergency psychiatric services are significant sequelae of abuse.

Prevalence

The prevalence of woman abuse among mental health clients is even greater than among medical patients, approaching half of all female inpatients. In addition, a substantial number of male patients in this population have also been abused by family members. Finally, a substantial number of both male and female inpatients have abused their partners.

Hilberman and Munson (75) found that 30 of 60 women referred for psychiatric consultation in a rural medical clinic were in relationships with batterers, although abuse had been previously identified as an issue for only four of the women. Approximately half of all female inpatients have been physically and/or sexually abused, more than twice the number of males who report abuse (33,61). Overall, according to Carmen (Hilberman) et al., 43 percent of the inpatients studied had histories of physical and sexual abuse, 90 percent by family members (33). Whereas men in that population were most likely to have been physically abused as teenagers by their fathers, women often were sexually as well as physically abused in childhood and as adults. Finally, Stark (8) reported that fully 25 percent of the women utilizing a psychiatric emergency service had a history of domestic violence.

Presenting Problems

Compared to nonbattered mental health patients, battered women are less likely to manifest psychotic illness, but more likely to carry a diagnosis of situational or personality disorder according to DSM-II (99) and to exhibit impaired self-esteem (33). Whereas battered women tend to direct anger inward, often in self-destructive ways, battered males (mainly adolescents) are more likely to channel self-hatred into aggression toward others (33). Still, in this highly disturbed population, there are no differences between battered and nonbattered groups on clinical scales of the Minnesota Multiphasic Personality Inventory (MMPI) or in the incidence of suicide attempts.

Among psychiatric emergency patients, alcoholism is twice as common among battered than nonbattered women (20% vs. 10%). Despite a marked absence of psychiatric disease, battered alcoholics had a mean rate of psychiatric emergency utilization that was three times greater than nonbattered alcoholics and a trauma history ten times greater (8).

Battered women have a significantly higher rate of psychiatric utilization than nonbattered women prior to the first reported abusive injury, which suggests that psychiatric illness may be the context for abuse in some instances. After abusive injury, utilization rises to 37 percent; 78 percent of the battered women who use psychiatric services following abuse have not done so previously (4,8). The most common diagnosis carried by abuse victims is depression (37%), but one abused woman in ten suffers a psychotic break (8). At the same time, battered women are also far more likely than others to be given a pseudopsychiatric label such as "hysteric," "hypochondriac," "crock," and so forth.

The Battering Syndrome

Although battering and abuse are sometimes used interchangeably, from the standpoint of health risks battering refers to the physical and psychosocial sequelae of woman abuse and includes a history of injury (often punctuated by sexual assault), general medical complaints, isolation and psychosocial problems that develop over time. In lieu of effective intervention, these sequelae have a cumulative cost and impact on health services that is far greater than the impact of abuse-related injury alone, often involving dozens, sometimes hundreds of medical and mental health visits. Indeed, recent evidence suggests that battering is a major cause of homelessness among women and children (100). The combination of assault and institutional victimization constitutes "the dual trauma" of battering, facilitates and extends male control over women's lives, and leads to an increasing sense of isolation, fear, entrapment, self-destructive behavior, and even homicidal rage among abused women. Although each of the problems associated with abuse may appear to have an independent etiology and although the multi-problem profile that often presents with abuse may seem intractable, the emergence of these problems only after a history of abuse and frustrated help-seeking is well established. This underscores the importance of early intervention at primary care sites as well as at each of the secondary treatment sites where the psychosocial consequences of living in a violent relationship are managed.

INTERVENTIONS TO PREVENT WOMAN BATTERING

This section outlines the current response to spouse abuse and the potential role of health providers in a multilevel (and multidisciplinary) prevention strategy.

Current Interventions

Preventing spouse abuse requires (1) protecting victims, (2) stopping violence, (3) expanding the resources and options available to victims and
assailants, (4) early identification and referral, and (5) public education.
Thus far, emphasis has been placed on shelter, police and legal action, and
legislation.

Federal and State Response

In the effort to prevent domestic violence, the Battered Women's Movement
has been unique in its community base, in the importance of abused women
in its development, and in its attempt to combine direct service to victims
with "empowerment." The emergence of almost 1,000 shelters for battered
women in the United States since the early 1970s has probably been the
single most important stimulus to the response of lawmakers, service providers, and researchers (101). In 1988 these shelters provided emergency
services to an cstimated 350,000 women.

State responses have emphasized legal reform, shelter funding, professional training, and the redirection of protective and human service resources. By 1988 the civil and criminal remedies available to abuse victims in
almost every state had improved, and 28 states mandated some form of
reporting from law enforcement and/or health services; many states
strongly urge or mandate police to arrest when there is evidence of injury or
other probable cause to believe a domestic assault has occurred.* A number
of states support shelters through special "add-ons" to the marriage license
fee, allocations through existing human service agencies, or broadened
definitions of how categorical aid, emergency housing, block grant, and
victim assistance funds will be spent. Several states have formed state-level
commissions (New York) or agencies (New Jersey) to oversee action on
domestic violence, including training for health, mental health, and social
service personnel. Recent state initiatives have extended training in domestic
violence to parole, probation and court staff, substance abuse counselors,
and child protective service workers. Interestingly, though battered women
comprise a significant percentage of the homeless population, funding and
service priorities in the area of homelessness rarely take this into account.

The federal response has primarily emphasized technical assistance and
research, though current legislation offers direct support to battered wom-
en's shelters. From 1974 until its closing, the Law Enforcement Assistance
Administration (LEAA) supported some direct services (including several
shelters) and court mediation programs for battered women. And Housing
and Urban Development (HUD) revisions in the Community Development
Block Grant guidelines permitted local purchase of shelters and other direct

*Common provisions of these measures are to (1) make spouse abuse a separate offense, (2)
make available pro se civil orders of protection and make violation of these orders a criminal
offense, (3) expand police arrest authority for misdemeanor assaults they do not witness, and
(4) provide police officers with liability immunity for good faith actions.

services. Meanwhile, after an unfavorable review of its child abuse program by the Office of Technical Assistance, the Department of Defense expanded its efforts to encompass spouse abuse and now offers comprehensive services for victims and assailants at major military installations. Health personnel play a key role in these programs. Following experimental police training programs, the Department of Justice funded pilot programs in several cities. Similarly, the National Institute of Justice is conducting a multisite study to assess findings from a Minneapolis experiment that arrest reduces the reoccurrence of abuse.

The U.S. Commission on Civil Rights held hearings on battered women in 1978. One outgrowth was the formation of the National Coalition Against Domestic Violence (NCADV), an umbrella organization representing state battered women's coalitions. NCADV was the first national organization to support shelter legislation and continues to coordinate shelter-oriented education and advocacy for battered women nationwide. To collect and disseminate information to service providers, President Carter established the Office of Domestic Violence (ODV) in 1979, but it was closed before Ronald Reagan took office. Although not a membership organization, the National Woman Abuse Prevention Project (NWAPP) combines elements of both NCADV and ODV, targeting shelter-oriented education to service providers, for example. Other national organizations representing women's interests have also contributed to increasing the visibility of battering, including the National Organization for Women (NOW) and the National Organization of Victim Advocates (NOVA). Meanwhile, National Institute of Mental Health (NIMH) divisions focusing on rape and on crime and delinquency supported a range of studies, meetings, and interventions, including a national survey of spouse abuse. More recently, an Attorney General's Task Force on Domestic Violence held hearings and issued a widely circulated report focusing on the need for a nationally coordinated criminal justice response to spouse abuse.

Three consecutive attempts to pass the Domestic Violence Assistance Act failed (1978, 1979, 1980), in part due to counterpressure from extreme conservatives, but a revised bill passed both houses in 1984, and six million dollars was appropriated. Some states can now fund shelter programs through federal victim compensation legislation.

The Medical Response

In the early 1970s, emergency service nurses in many hospitals established protocols to provide intensive crisis intervention for sexual assault victims. Building on this base and following the lead of the Ambulatory Nursing Department of the Brigham and Women's Hospital in Boston, several hospitals introduced domestic violence protocols. The potential development of a database indicating the significance of abuse for women's health stimulated the Centers for Disease Control (CDC) in Atlanta to have its Violence Epidemiology Branch assess the feasibility of a national domestic violence surveillance system, to encourage a focus on battering by projects in trauma registry and injury prevention and control, and, most recently, to determine whether medical education has developed domestic violence curricula (102). Meanwhile, New York and New Jersey have developed model protocols for hospitals and Connecticut contracts with the Domestic Violence Training Project (DVTP) specifically to train its health providers. Maine, Ohio, Massachusetts, Texas, Washington, and other states, have sponsored major training efforts directed at nursing, social service, and emergency medical staff. The Double Jeopardy project in Los Angeles County has highlighted links between alcohol and violence, an issue that has also been the focus of training efforts in New Jersey, New York, and Connecticut. The relation between domestic violence and health has been a major focus for a national women's nursing network.

Hoping to provide national leadership in the health sector, C. Everett Koop, then surgeon general, sponsored an unprecedented Workshop on Violence and Public Health in Leesburg, Virginia, in October 1985. This was followed by regional conferences focused on similar themes and, most recently, by a campaign by the American College of Obstetricians and Gynecologists to help physicians detect and assist victims of domestic violence. The impact of battering on poor outcomes in pregnancy has been acknowledged in two recent initiatives, a training program targeting maternal and child health providers funded by the March of Dimes and a massive outreach program on domestic violence to the membership of the American College of Obstetricians and Gynecologists. In October 1989 the American Medical Association held an important conference on family violence that was co-sponsored by 50 medical, legal, and social service organizations. The hospital sector has been slow to respond to these initiatives, however, as have the primary care and mental health sectors to which battered women turn for most of their care. Health researchers have also been slow to respond. Indicative of this lack of response is a recent survey, published in *Injury in America* (103), prepared by the National Research Council and the Institute of Medicine. This survey dismisses violence, homicide, and assault with a sentence or two and completely fails to mention battering, the major source of injury to women.

A New Health Perspective

The knowledge base exists for a coordinated response to spouse abuse by the health care community. As we have seen, however, the current medical response may even contribute to the problem through a failure to identify the problem or to accurately assess its significance. For the following reasons, the traditional medical model of disease is inadequate:

1. It misses or greatly undervalues the psychological and social costs of abuse. Only when these costs are considered along with the costs of injury can the full importance of battering and spouse abuse be appreciated.

2. In its emphasis on biology, personality, or risk behaviors, the traditional medical model underplays the complex social origins of spouse abuse. The "political" model of spouse abuse, which emphasizes the use of violence to enforce inequality, finds stronger support than alternative explanations highlighting pathology, risk behaviors, or stress. Closing what Reiker and Carmen (104) call the "gender gap" in medical and psychiatric services requires that clinicians base identification on patient self-assessment, that discrete presentations be seen in the context of a woman's entire history, and that clinicians stop blaming abuse on its victims.

3. The traditional disease model has generated notions of prevention that must be changed. Traditional methods of screening for susceptibility and/or managing risk behaviors have little bearing on spouse abuse. Instead, interventions must target social behaviors and the social environment; health providers must form working alliances with community-based services (such as shelters) and with disciplines outside health (including social science); and an emphasis should be placed on nonmedical policies and interventions that can reduce violence and improve health. We term this approach complex social prevention. This should include—but not be limited to—working alliances at the national and local level between major health care providers and state shelter coalitions and national organizations representing services for spouse abuse victims such as NCADV and NWAPP.

Recommended Interventions

This section outlines a multilevel (and multidisciplinary) strategy to prevent battering and substantially reduce spouse abuse. Complex social prevention involves broad changes in our overall approach to violence and is designed to reduce the use of violence to perpetuate gender inequality in intimate relations. Primary prevention involves intervening in cases of potential battering before a pattern of victimization is established. Secondary prevention attempts to minimize the consequences and costs of battering by providing its victims with appropriate support.

Complex Social Prevention

These interventions are designed to change the social, cultural, and physical contexts most likely to evoke violence among social partners. The underlying premise of these interventions is that nonmedical policies and practices may have the greatest bearing on health.

1. *Increase our knowledge of the causes of spouse abuse and the interventions that most effectively prevent it.* Knowledge of what causes spouse abuse or why woman abuse typically leads to battering is far less extensive than knowledge of the scope and consequences of domestic violence. Moreover, what studies there are highlight interpersonal factors rather than the

structural factors implicated by the gender-politics model. There is a need for critical evaluation of existing services and interventions (105) and for controlled comparisons of various interventions such as the Minneapolis police experiment.

2. *Give national recognition to the criminal nature of spouse abuse with particular emphasis on its health consequences for women.* National leadership from the political and health communities should establish that physical safety in social relationships is a basic health right. The initiatives by the surgeon general and the Centers for Disease Control are steps in this direction.

3. *Decrease the cultural acceptance of violence against vulnerable groups.* There is widespread tolerance for violence among and/or against certain disadvantaged or vulnerable groups (women, blacks, teenagers, children) based on cultural stereotypes and theories of diminished responsibility for impulsive behavior. Public health education should target beliefs that view interpersonal violence as a legitimate response to jealousy or economic hardship, for example, as well as explanations that blame or otherwise denigrate the victims of violence. Such education is an important component of a successful domestic violence prevention program in Duluth, Minnesota.

4. *Support the empowerment of women by expanding their social and economic options.* Millions of women become entrapped in violent homes because of limited social and economic opportunities. Many victims of abuse are denied effective access to resources to which they are legally entitled, including health care, by discrimination based on race, income, educational deficits, or gender. Whereas equal access is an important goal, role change may be more important. This entails supporting women's independence from traditional family responsibilities (such as child and health care); supporting single family heads through daycare, low-cost housing, educational opportunity, and increased aid to dependent children (ADC); and fostering the assumption of greater homemaking and child-care responsibilities by men. Empowerment also means greater decision-making power for abused women in health and other service settings. Such support is particularly important during the abuse victim's transition to independent living.

5. *Make spouse abuse prevention a major priority for all human resource and public health funding.* The time has come to "mainstream" abuse by making it an issue in every area of service that affects women's lives, for example, in housing, job training, and family planning. To do this requires sensitizing personnel in local, state, and federal agencies to abuse and acknowledging abuse as a high priority in federal, state, and local grant programs, including funds for community mental health and neighborhood health centers and the public health components of the block grant. Objectives should include communitywide (or institution-based) surveillance of spouse abuse; programs to reduce the isolation of female heads of house-

hold; campaigns against misogyny in the media; elimination of those facets of public policy that reinforce women's dependence on the male head of household; support for neighborhood-based mediation programs; and increased housing, education, and employment options, particularly for women with children.

6. *Support more flexible role models for women and men.* Traditional role stereotypes of males and females are implicated in the enormous morbidity from domestic violence. Based in public education about these hazards, new models of role flexibility should be promoted that emphasize shared decision-making, nonviolent means of self-expression and dispute settlement, and women's right to resist male violence and control. To fulfill new roles will require material incentives such as meaningful roles for unemployed men and paternity leave.

Primary Prevention

These interventions are designed to prevent battering by enabling health institutions to respond more effectively to interpersonal conflict (and abuse) before it escalates.

1. *Establish and implement model protocols for the early identification and referral of abuse victims in health settings.* Evidence suggests that abuse can be readily identified—and battering prevented—by combining an adult trauma history with direct questioning about violence and control in the home. Emphasizing early identification, supportive education, effective referral, and ongoing support and follow-up for abused women at primary care sites could eventually reduce the prevalence of abusive injury by up to 75 percent and dramatically impact the incidence of female alcoholism, child abuse, female suicide attempts, and mental illness.

2. *Introduce model curricula on spouse abuse and gender bias into the professional education, training, and continuing education of health and social service providers.* In an effort to close the "gender gap" in medical and mental health education, provider organizations should work with organizations representing battered women to introduce relevant materials on spouse abuse into the regular training of all health and social service providers, including doctors, nurses, emergency medical technicians (EMTs), social workers, substance abuse counselors, ministers, psychologists, school counselors, and criminal justice groups.

3. *Develop and distribute public information on spouse abuse and available services for media.* The majority of women at risk for abuse may not view their problems as health-related. In conjunction with NCADV, NWAPP, and state coalitions representing battered women, the Public Health Service and relevant state agencies should develop and distribute public service announcements highlighting the illegality of abuse, its dangers to women and children, and available services for victims.

Secondary Prevention

These interventions are designed to reduce the evolution from abuse to woman battering and the suffering associated with established patterns of spouse abuse.

1. *Support the development of spouse abuse protocols in secondary treatment sites dealing with rape, alcohol and drug abuse, suicide prevention, emergency psychiatric problems, child abuse, and the homeless.* Despite the fact that battering is a major contributor to attempted suicide, female alcoholism, child abuse, homelessness, and emergency psychiatric problems, programs dealing with these issues rarely identify male violence as an issue or target its elimination. National influence should be exerted to bring violence to the attention of service providers in these areas and to encourage innovative programs that accommodate the special needs of battering victims.

2. *Extend the range of options available to battered women.* As the first-line protection for abuse victims, community-based shelters should receive all possible recognition and support from national health care provider organizations. Survivors of battering should be directly involved in professional training and education. In addition, the need for emergency housing and other vital resources should be met by providing safe wards in local health institutions; ensuring priority status for abuse victims in public housing; creating second-stage housing during the transition from shelter to independent living; making abuse victims automatically eligible for disaster relief, Social Security Insurance (SSI), ADC, Medicaid, and other public assistance programs; and giving victims priority status in Head Start and job training.

3. *Expand the options available to violent men.* Health and social services in this country are largely used by and oriented towards women. Abusive males appear to respond well to behavior-oriented counseling (particularly as an alternative to jail), which emphasizes the inappropriateness of traditional male roles, respect for female independence, taking responsibility for violent acts, and learning nonviolent means of responding to interpersonal tension. Program models include EMERGE in Boston, AMEND in Denver, Brother-to-Brother in Rhode Island, the open-ended program developed by Anne Gagnley at the Veterans Administration (VA) in Seattle, and the batterers' program developed by Ellen Pence in conjunction with the Family Court in Duluth, Minnesota.

ANNOTATED BIBLIOGRAPHY

Bowker LH. Ending the violence. Holmes Beach, FL: Learning Publications, 1986.
    This volume assesses strategies women have used to end violence or escape violent relationships. It offers important practical suggestions for social service providers in health care settings.

Dobash RE, Dobash RP. Violence against wives. New York: Free Press, 1979.

> The authors present a theoretical and historical overview of wife abuse and an excellent critical summary of existing approaches to the problem. They trace the victims of abuse through the life-cycle and highlight the situational dynamics of battering relationships. The critical discussion of health and social services is particularly astute.

Finkelhor D et al., eds. The dark side of families: Current family violence research. Beverly Hills, CA: Sage, 1983.

> This collection from the First National Research Conference on Domestic Violence includes important critical articles on husband abuse, on maternal child abuse, on public attitudes towards domestic violence, and on the response to spouse abuse by health providers.

Reiker PP, Carmen (Hilberman) E. The gender gap in psychotherapy: Social realities and psychological processes. New York: Plenum, 1984.

> Drawing on the extensive research reconceptualizing women's psychology, the articles collected in this volume assess the effect of social structure on psychological processes, review the clinical consequences of gender inequality, and trace the implications for treatment and professional education. The book includes several important articles on battered women by Elaine Carmen (Hilberman).

Schecter S. Women and male violence. Boston: South End Press, 1982.

> This comprehensive history of the Battered Women's Movement by an important figure in its development highlights the philosophy and practice of shelters and some of the key controversies and dilemmas confronting the shelter movement, and presents a critical view of male violence from a feminist perspective.

Stark E, Flitcraft A. Women and children at risk: A feminist perspective on child abuse. Int J Health Services 1988; 18:97–118.

> The authors critically review the response of the child abuse establishment to the discovery of woman battering and assess evidence that violence against women originates in the family of origin. They present data from a hospital-based study showing that male violence against women is a major precipitant of child abuse.

Stark E, Flitcraft A, Frazier W. Medicine and patriarchal violence: The social construction of a "private" event. Int J Health Services 1979; 9:461–493.

> Starting with a month's sample of women using a major metropolitan emergency service, the authors develop a technique for identifying abuse in the medical record, describe the health consequences and stages of battering, and argue that the current medical response contributes to the development of this syndrome.

Straus M, Gelles R, Steinmetz SK. Behind closed doors: A survey of family violence in America. New York: Doubleday, 1980.

> The only representative national survey of spouse abuse in America is reported at length in this volume. The evidence encompasses a range of forceful acts—from sibling fights through severe violence—and bears on a number of explanatory theories, including the intergenerational transmission of violence.

REFERENCES

1. Straus M, Gelles R, Steinmetz SK. Behind closed doors: A survey of family violence in America. New York: Doubleday, 1980.
2. Berk RA, Berk SF, Loseke DR, Rauma D. Mutual combat and other family violence myths. In: Finkelhor D et al., eds. The dark side of families: Current family violence research. Beverly Hills, CA: Sage, 1983.

3. Stark E, Flitcraft A, Frazier W. Medicine and patriarchal violence: The social construction of a "private" event. Int J Health Services 1979; 9:461–493.
4. Stark E, Flitcraft A, et al. Wife abuse in the medical setting: An introduction for health personnel. Monograph #7. Washington, DC: Office of Domestic Violence, 1981.
5. O'Leary KD. Physical aggression between spouses: A social learning theory perspective. In: Van Hasselt VB, Morrison RL, Bellack AS, Hersen M, eds. Handbook of family violence. New York: Plenum, 1988; 31–56.
6. Gauquin DA. Spouse abuse: Data from the National Crime Survey. Victimology 1977–78; 2:632–643.
7. Walker L. The battered woman. New York: Harper & Row, 1979.
8. Stark E. The battering syndrome: Social knowledge, social therapy and the abuse of women (dissertation). SUNY-Binghamton, 1984.
9. Stark E, Flitcraft A. Violence among intimates: An epidemiological review. In: Hasselt VN et al., eds. Handbook of family violence. New York: Plenum, 1988; 293–318.
10. Stark E, Flitcraft A. Social knowledge, social policy and the abuse of women. In: Finkelhor D et al., eds. The dark side of families. Beverly Hills, CA: Sage, 1983.
11. Teske RHC, Parker ML. Spouse abuse in Texas: A study of women's attitudes and experiences. Huntsville, TX: Criminal Justice Center, Sam Houston State University, 1983.
12. Cambell JC. Testimony: Select committee to study the need for availability of funding for domestic violence and rape crisis services in Pennsylvania. Harrisburg, PA, Feb. 21, 1990.
13. Rosenberg ML, Stark E, Zahn MA. Interpersonal violence: Homicide and spouse abuse. In: Last JM, ed. Maxcy-Rosenau public health and preventive medicine, 12th ed. New York: Appleton-Century Crofts, 1985.
14. Hornung CA, McCullough BC, Sugimoto T. Status relationships in marriage: Risk factors in spouse abuse. J Marriage Family 1981; 43:675–692.
15. Szinovacz ME. Using couple data as a methodological tool: The case of marital violence. J Marriage Family 1983; 45:633–644.
16. Meredith WH, Abbott DA, Adams SL. Family violence: Its relation to marital and parental satisfaction and family strengths. J Family Violence 1986; 1:299–305.
17. Straus MA, Gelles RJ. Violence in American families. In: Chilman CC, Cox F, Nunnaly E, eds. Families in trouble. Beverly Hills, CA: Sage, 1987.
18. Schulman MA. Survey of spousal violence against women in Kentucky. Harris Study #792701, 1979.
19. Genteman KM. Attitudes of North Carolina women toward the acceptance and causes of wife beating. Nashville. Paper presented at the meeting of the Southeastern Women's Studies Association, 1980.
20. Flitcraft A. Battered women: An emergency room epidemiology with a description of a clinical syndrome and critique of present therapeutics. Doctoral thesis, New Haven, Yale University School of Medicine, 1977.
21. Christiano M et al. Battered women: A concern for the medical profession. Connecticut Med 1986; 50:99–103.
22. Anwar R. Woman abuse: Retrospective review of all female trauma presenting to the emergency room. Philadelphia: Medical College of Pennsylvania, 1976.
23. McCleer SV, Anwar R. A study of women presenting in an emergency department. Am J Public Health 1989; 79:65–67.

24. Kurz D, Stark E. Health education and feminist strategy: The case of woman abuse. In: Yllo K, Bograd M, eds. Feminist perspectives on wife abuse. Beverly Hills, CA: Sage, 1988.

25. Denzin N. Toward a phenomenology of domestic, family violence. AJS 1984; 90:483–513.

26. Wardell L, Gillespie DL, Hansen KV. Science and violence against wives. In: Finkelhor D, Gelles RJ, Hotaling GT, Straus MA, eds. The dark side of families: Current family violence research. Beverly Hills, CA: Sage, 1983; 69–84.

27. Breines W, Gordon L. The new scholarship on family violence. Signs: J Women Culture Society 1983; 8:490–531.

28. Kantor GK, Straus M. The drunken bum theory of wife beating. Social Problems (in press).

29. Cambell JC, Humphreys JH. Nursing care of victims of family violence. Reston, VA: Reston, 1984.

30. Walker LEA. Psychological causes of family violence. In: Lystad M, ed. Violence in the home: Interdisciplinary perspectives. New York: Bruner/Mazel, 1986; 71–97.

31. Bersani CA, Chen H. Sociological perspectives in family violence. In: Van Hasselt VB, Morrison RL, Bellack AS, Hersen M, eds. Handbook of family violence. New York: Plenum, 1988; 57–88.

32. McCleer SV. Psychoanalytic perspectives on family violence. In: Van Hasselt VB, Morrison R, Bellack AS, Hersen M, eds. Handbook of family violence. New York: Plenum, 1988; 11–31.

33. Carmen (Hilberman) E, Rieker P, Mills T. Victims of violence and psychiatric illness. Am J Psychiatry 1984; 141:378–383.

34. Stark E, Flitcraft A. Woman-battering, child abuse and social heredity: What is the relationship? In: Johnson N, ed. Marital violence. Sociological Review Monograph #31. London: Routledge & Kegan Paul, 1985.

35. Gayford JJ. Wife battering: A preliminary survey of 100 cases. Br Med J 1975; 1:194–197.

36. Stark E, Flitcraft A. Women and children at risk: A feminist perspective on child abuse. Int J Health Services 1988; 18:97–118.

37. Baum A, Fleming R, Singer JE. Coping with victimization by technological disaster. J Social Issues 1983; 39:119–140.

38. Bulman R, Wortman C. Attributions of blame and coping in the "real world": Severe accident victims react to their lot. J Personality Social Psychology 1977; 35:351–363.

39. Miller DT, Porter CA. Self-blame in victims of violence. J Social Issues 1983; 39:139–152.

40. Cambell JC. A test of two explanatory models of women's response to battering. Nursing Res 1989; 38:18–24.

41. Stark E, Flitcraft A. Personal power and institutional victimization: Treating the dual trauma of woman battering. In: Ochberg F, ed. Post traumatic therapy. New York: Bruner/Mazel, 1987.

42. Kaufman J, Zigler E. Do abused children become abusive parents? Unpublished paper, Bush Child Study Center, Yale University, 1986.

43. Makepeace JM. The severity of courtship violence injuries and the effectiveness of individual precautions. In: Hotaling G et al., eds. Family abuse and its consequences: New directions in research. Beverly Hills, CA: Sage, 1988; 297–311.

44. Gil D. Violence against children: Physical child abuse in the United States. Cambridge, MA: Harvard University Press, 1973.
45. Finn J. The stresses and coping behavior of battered women. Social Casework 1985: 341–349.
46. Casanave NA, Straus MA. Race, class, network embeddedness and family violence: A search for potent support systems. J Comparative Family Studies 1979; 10:281–299.
47. Brown GW, Harris T. Social origins of depression—a study of psychiatric disorder in women. London: Tavistock, 1978.
48. Contoni L. Clinical issues in domestic violence. Social Casework 1981; 62:3–12.
49. Graff TT. Personality characteristics of battered women. Dissertation Abstracts International 1980; 40(7B):3395.
50. Telch CF, Lindquist CU. Violent versus nonviolent couples: A comparison of patterns. Psychotherapy 1984; 21:242–248.
51. Star B. Comparing battered and nonbattered women. Victimology 1978; 3:32–44.
52. Frieze IH. Causal attributions as mediators of battered women's response to battering. (Grant #1 R01 MH30193). Washington, DC: National Institute of Mental Health, 1980.
53. Giles-Simms J. Wife-battering: A systems theory approach. New York: Guilford Press, 1983.
54. Walker L. The battered woman syndrome study. In: Finkelhor D et al., eds. The dark side of families. Beverly Hills, CA: Sage, 1983.
55. Petro J et al. Wife abuse. JAMA 1978; 240:240–241.
56. Gelles R. The violent home. Beverly Hills, CA: Sage, 1974.
57. Steinmetz SK. Occupational environment in relation to physical punishment and dogmatism. In: Straus M, Steinmetz S, eds. Violence in the family. New York: Harper & Row, 1974.
58. Peterson R. Social class, social learning and wife abuse. Social Service Rev 1980; 54:390–406.
59. Hotaling GT, Sugerman DB. An identification of risk factors. In: Domestic violence surveillance system feasibility study, phase I report. Atlanta: Centers for Disease Control, 1984.
60. Dvoskin JA. Battered women—an epidemiological study of spousal violence. Ph.D. dissertation, University of Arizona, 1981.
61. Post RD, Willett AB, Franks RD, et al. A preliminary report on the prevalence of domestic violence among psychiatric inpatients. Am J Psychiatry 1980; 137:974–975.
62. Garbarino J, Sherman D. High-risk families and high-risk neighborhoods. Child Dev 1980; 51:188–198.
63. Bowen G. Spouse abuse: Incidence and dynamics. Military Family 1984; 33:667–682.
64. Helton AS. Battering during pregnancy: A prevalence study in a metropolitan area. M.S. thesis, Denton, College of Nursing, Texas Woman's University, 1985.
65. Hillard PJA. Physical abuse in pregnancy. Obst Gynecol 1985; 66:185–190.
66. Okun L. Woman abuse: Facts replacing myths. Albany: SUNY Press, 1986.
67. Byles JA. Violence, alcohol problems and other problems in disintegrating families. J Studies Alcohol 1979; 39.
68. Coleman DH, Straus M. Alcohol use and family violence. In: Gottheil E,

Druley KA, Skoloda TE, Waxman HM, eds. Alcohol, drug abuse and aggression. Springfield, IL: Charles C Thomas, 1983; 104–124.

69. Orne TC, Rimmer J. Alcoholism and child abuse: A review. J Studies Alcohol 1980; 42.

70. McClintock FH. Criminological aspects of family violence. In: Martin JP, ed. Violence and the family. New York: Wiley, 1978.

71. Bard M, Zacker J. Assaultiveness and alcohol use in family disputes: Police perceptions. Criminology 1974; 12:281–292.

72. Richardson DC, Cambell JL. Alcohol and wife abuse: The effect of alcohol on attributions of blame for wife abuse. Personality Social Psychol Bull 1980; 6:51–56.

73. Corenblum B. Reactions to alcohol-related marital violence. J Studies on Alcohol 1983; 44(4):665–674.

74. Rosenbaum A, O'Leary P. Marital violence: Characteristics of abusive couples. J Consulting Clin Psychology 1981; 41:63–71.

75. Hilberman E, Munson K. Sixty battered women. Victimology 1977-78; 2:460–470.

76. Pahl J. The general practitioner and the problem of battered women. J Med Ethics 1979; 5:117–123.

77. Straus MA, Gelles RJ. Physical violence in American families: Risk factors and adaptation to violence in 8,145 families. New Brunswick, NJ: Transaction Books, 1989.

78. Nisonoff L, Bitman I. Spouse abuse: Incidence and relationship to selected demographic variables. Victimology 1979; 4:131–140.

79. Steinmetz SK. The battered husband syndrome. Victimology 1977-78; 2:499–509.

80. Klaus PA, Rand MR. Family violence. Special report by the Bureau of Justice Statistics. Washington, DC: US Dept. of Justice, 1984.

81. Russell D. The prevalence and impact of marital rape in San Francisco. Paper presented the meeting of the American Sociological Association, 1980.

82. Russell D. Rape in marriage. New York: Macmillan, 1982.

83. Bogal-Allbritten RB, Allbritten B. The hidden victims: Premarital abuse among college students. Anaheim, CA. Paper presented at meeting of American Psychological Association, 1983.

84. Murphy JE. Date abuse and forced intercourse among college students. Durham, NH. Paper presented at the Second National Family Violence Research Conference, 1984.

85. Kurz D. Responses to battered women: Resistance to medicalization. Social Problems 1988; 34:501–513.

86. Appleton W. The battered woman syndrome. Ann Emergency Med 1980; 9:84–91.

87. Gerson LW. Alcohol related acts of violence: Who was drinking and where the acts occurred. J Studies Alcohol 1978; 39:1294–1296.

88. Pagelow MD. Preliminary report on battered women. Boston. Paper presented at the Second International Symposium on Victimology, 1976.

89. Roper M, Flitcraft A, Frazier W. Rape and battering: A pilot study. Department of Surgery, Yale Medical School, 1979.

90. Cohn DA et al. The psychological adjustment of school-aged children of battered women: A preliminary look. Durham, NH. Paper presented at the Second National Conference for Family Violence Researchers, 1984.

91. Levine M. Interparental violence and its effect on the children: A study of 50 families in general practice. Med Sci Law 1975; 15:172.
92. Brown AJ, Pelcovitz D, Kaplan S. Clinical witnesses of family violence: A study of psychological correlates. Anaheim, CA. Paper presented at meeting of American Psychological Association, 1983.
93. Stewart MA, deBlois CS. Wife abuse among families attending a child psychiatry clinic. J Am Acad Child Psychiatry 1981; 20:845.
94. Bowker LH. On the relationship between wife-beating and child abuse. In: Yllo K, Bograd M, eds. Feminist perspectives on wife abuse. Beverly Hills, CA: Sage, 1988.
95. Martin J. Maternal and paternal abuse of children: Theoretical and research perspectives. In: Finkelhor D et al., eds. The dark side of families: Current family violence research. Beverly Hills, CA: Sage, 1983.
96. Bergman A, Larsen RM, Mueller B. Changing spectrum of serious child abuse. Pediatrics 1986; 77:113–116.
97. American Humane Society. National analysis of official child neglect and abuse reporting. Denver: AHA, 1978.
98. Baher E et al. At risk: An account of the work of the battered child research department, NSPCC. Boston: Routledge & Kegan Paul, 1976.
99. Back SM, Post RD, D'Arcy H. A comparison of battered and nonbattered female psychiatric patients. Montreal. Paper presented at meeting of American Psychological Association, 1980.
100. Bassuck EL, Rosenberg L. Why does family homelessness occur? A case-control study. AVPH 1988; 28:783–788.
101. Schechter S. Women and male violence. Boston: South End Press, 1982.
102. Centers for Disease Control. Education in adult domestic violence: Current trends in U.S. and Canadian medical schools, 1987–88. Morbidity and Mortality Weekly Report 1989; 38(2):17–19.
103. National Research Council and the Institute of Medicine. Injury in America: A continuing public health problem. Washington, DC: National Academy Press, 1985.
104. Reiker PP, Carmen (Hilberman) E. The gender gap in psychotherapy: Social realities and psychological processes. New York: Plenum, 1984.
105. Bowker LH. Ending the violence. Holmes Beach, FL: Learning Publications, 1986.

7

Domestic Violence
Against the Elderly

KARL PILLEMER AND SUSAN FRANKEL

This chapter provides a comprehensive review of research on domestic elder abuse. First, definitional problems are reviewed, and it is asserted that no widely accepted definition of the problem exists. For the purpose of clarity, this chapter focuses on physical violence against the elderly by family members. Second, existing data sources about elder abuse are described. Sources fall into three major categories: surveys, case-control studies, and other sources. Third, a theoretical framework is proposed that stresses five potential causes of elder abuse: intraindividual dynamics, intergenerational transmission of violent behavior, dependency and exchange relations between abuser and abused, external stress, and social isolation. Fourth, consequences of elder abuse are discussed; lack of data, however, prevents specification of the nature and extent of such effects. Finally, potential interventions to assist elder abuse victims and their families are reviewed. The overall evidence in this area suggests a move away from an emphasis on mandatory reporting laws and adult protective services to a focus on developing a comprehensive community-based service system for elders and their families.

STATEMENT OF THE PROBLEM

The problem of elder abuse and neglect first came to the public's attention in the early 1980s. Reports of elder abuse have appeared in many mass media publications and on national television. In the midst of discussions and controversies about elder abuse, many persons professionally and personally concerned about the elderly find themselves confused about the issue.

How much elder abuse is there? What causes elder abuse? Who is most likely to be affected?

Such questions have been difficult to answer because very little was known about elder abuse. Methodologically sound research on elder abuse has been extremely scarce. With a few exceptions, most studies on the topic have been so seriously flawed that they are unreliable. Barriers to effective utilization of research have included use of vague and inconsistent definitions of elder abuse, exclusive reliance on professional assessments, and absence of control groups.

Recently, however, our knowledge about elder abuse has increased somewhat. Researchers have begun to employ more rigorous research designs, and policy analysts have subjected elder abuse intervention programs to careful scrutiny. This chapter reviews research efforts to understand the incidence and causes of elder abuse, and highlights major intervention strategies.

Definitions

A major difficulty in analyzing results from previous research on elder abuse and neglect results from the poor definition of the term elder abuse. Many researchers refer to an entire range of problems the elderly can experience as *abuse*, including lack of proper housing, untreated medical conditions, and lack of social services. Furthermore, most studies are weakened by their undifferentiated treatment of various types of abuse and neglect: they lump all forms of mistreatment together, despite evidence that the forms of abuse and neglect differ substantially (1,2).

Thus there is no consensus as to how elder abuse should be properly defined. Researchers have varied widely in the way they define the term, frequently using confusing and unclear definitions. This definitional confusion makes results from many studies nearly impossible to interpret. Examples of this definitional inconsistency can be seen by examining three recent studies.

In a study of abusive and nonabusive relationships, Phillips (3) used the following dimensions to define abuse: physical abuse, physical neglect, emotional abuse, emotional neglect, emotional deprivation, sexual exploitation and assault, verbal assault, medical neglect, material abuse, neglect of the environment and violation of rights. In contrast, Bristowe and Collins (4) used only four categories of maltreatment: passive neglect, active neglect, physical abuse, and verbal abuse. Similarly, Pillemer and Finkelhor (5) focused on three forms of abuse: physical abuse, psychological abuse, and neglect.

Beyond such obvious differences, there are many other types of definitional inconsistencies. For example, financial exploitation has been included in several studies and excluded from others. Similarly, behaviors defined as psychological abuse differ among studies. For example, repeated insults and threats have been classified as psychological abuse (3), verbal abuse (4), and as verbal assault (3). Finally, it is difficult to know how some researchers differentiate abuse from neglect. Some researchers distinguish types of neglect (e.g., active vs. passive, or physical vs. emotional), whereas others maintain neglect as a single category. As these examples indicate, the lack of uniformity and agreement makes it difficult to compare and analyze research findings. Several reviewers of the elder abuse literature have provided useful critical analyses of the definitional issue (1,6–10).

The development of better definitions of maltreatment of the elderly has become a high priority for researchers. In particular, it has become critical to differentiate among various types of maltreatment. Pedrick-Cornell and Gelles (1) have noted that acts of commission differ substantially from acts of omission in the characteristics of both the perpetrator and the victim. Evidence for this point comes from a project that evaluated different intervention programs for elder abuse and neglect. In this project, Wolf and Pillemer (11) differentiated abuse and neglect into five distinct categories: physical abuse, psychological abuse, material abuse, active neglect, and passive neglect. Further, they provided careful operational definitions for each type of abuse and neglect they described. They found that the characteristics of abusers and victims differed substantially among the abuse types.

Recently, Johnson (12) proposed an innovative approach to the definitional problem. In an attempt to incorporate all circumstances that constitute elder neglect, Johnson developed a four-stage definition: (1) conceptualization of the variable, (2) specification of behavioral manifestations, (3) measurement of observable events, and (4) separation of the act from the cause (p. 169). Whereas this four-stage approach may be a useful paradigm for researchers, practitioners need succinct, clear, operational definitions, and may find such an approach to be too all-encompassing (13, p. 13).

It is at present impossible to resolve the definitional disarray, although several reviews of previous research help to clarify basic definitions. First, all discussions of elder abuse include physical violence. There seems to be consensus among researchers and practitioners that physical assault against an elder constitutes abusive behavior. Second, most of the research literature includes a category of psychological or emotional abuse. Although these terms are often vaguely defined, psychological abuse must be included in any definition of elder mistreatment. Third, material abuse involves situations in which an elder's property or financial resources have been stolen or misused. Finally, the category of neglect appears in many studies, although there is not full agreement about how to define neglect. There appears to be general agreement that the intentional failure of a clearly designated caregiver to meet the needs of an elder constitutes neglect. Fulmer and Ashley (8), however, point out the difficulties in differentiating between the presence and absence of this form of maltreatment.

This chapter responds to the themes of this volume by focusing on *violence* against the elderly (persons 65 and older) in domestic settings. Whereas there continues to be some debate over the precise definitions of a "violent act," we have chosen to follow the simple and clear definition of

Straus, Gelles, and Steinmetz (14) who define violence as "an act carried out with the intention or perceived intention of causing physical pain or injury to another person." In this chapter the terms *elder abuse, elder mistreatment*, and *elder maltreatment* are used interchangeably.

DATA SOURCES

Research on the extent of elder abuse has been inconsistent because of the limited sources of data on the problem. The few studies conducted in the late 1970s and early 1980s were small, nonrandom, and largely exploratory in nature. Researchers have not utilized data sources similar to those that have been used in analyzing other forms of family violence (e.g., state statistics, emergency room records, or police reports). In this section, three sources of existing data are discussed: surveys, case-control studies, and other sources. One disclaimer is necessary at the outset of this review. As in any other field in which the knowledge base is rapidly growing, it is impossible to keep abreast of every new development, and there may be a number of relevant studies that have not yet come to our attention. In this chapter, greater attention is given to the more recent research studies. Several good review articles have been written in which the earlier studies on elder abuse have been discussed at greater length (7,9,10). Our goal is to identify examples of different approaches to the study of elder abuse rather than present an exhaustive review.

Surveys

Two basic designs have been employed in elder abuse surveys: random sample surveys and surveys of clinical professionals who have contact with elder abuse cases. Until recently, surveys of professionals have been the most frequently used research strategy.

Random Sample Surveys
One of the earliest random sample elder abuse surveys was conducted in 1979 by Block and Sinnott (15). This survey indicated that approximately 4 percent of the elderly are abused. The researchers mailed survey questionnaires to three different groups in the Washington, D.C. area: community agencies, a random sample of elderly persons living in the community, and health and human service professionals. These sources were questioned about a range of types of elder maltreatment, including physical, financial, and emotional abuse and neglect.

The findings from this study have been widely cited in the literature despite very serious methodological limitations. First, the response rate was low: only one agency in 24 responded, as did only 16 percent of the elderly and 31 percent of professionals. Second, the sample was very small (N = 73). Third, the survey asked about knowledge of abuse, rather than the actual experience of it. Finally, this survey was confined to the District of Columbia and its results cannot be generalized to the nation as a whole.

In contrast, a very low estimate of elder abuse comes from a survey conducted by Gioglio and Blakemore (16). This study was one of the first surveys of elder abuse and neglect based on a random probability sample of a state's population. A structured questionnaire was administered to a random sample of 324 elderly New Jersey residents to determine the extent of elder abuse. Only five persons reported some form of maltreatment. Projecting this figure to the entire noninstitutionalized elderly population of New Jersey, Gioglio and Blakemore estimated that 1 percent of the state's elderly population, or 8,000 persons, would report having been victimized.

There are problems with this survey as well. Only one of the five cases involved physical maltreatment; the other four were cases of financial exploitation. Moreover, the New Jersey study did not use very precise measures of abuse and relied on volunteer interviewers.

A more reliable survey, recently conducted by Pillemer and Finkelhor (17), attempted to assess the scope and nature of maltreatment of the elderly occurring in the community at large, including unreported and undetected elder abuse. The study was designed as a stratified random sample of all community-dwelling elderly persons (65 or older) in the Boston metropolitan area. In-person or telephone interviews were conducted with 2,020 elderly persons. Using a variety of measures, the survey inquired about respondents' personal experiences of three types of maltreatment: physical violence, chronic verbal aggression, and neglect by family members and other persons close to them. The authors estimated that between 2.5 percent and 3.9 percent of Boston area elderly persons had been maltreated in one or more of these three ways. If a national sample were to find a similar rate, it would indicate between 701,000 and 1,093,560 abused elders in the nation as a whole.

A nationwide survey of prevalence and circumstances of elder abuse in Canada (18) completed in 1989 found rates of elder abuse very similar to the Boston study, although some differences in study definitions existed. For comparable types of abuse, however, lower rates were found in Canada. These findings are consistent with the fact that violence rates in general are lower in Canada than in the United States.

These general population studies indicate that the extent of elder abuse may be less than previously suspected. Random sample surveys of the elderly population allow for a more accurate assessment of the rate of elder abuse. Such assessment is necessary in order to respond to the needs of victims and their families. A national survey is greatly needed to estimate rates of maltreatment for the United States as a whole.

Surveys of Professionals
The most common type of study performed and cited has been the survey of professionals who work with the elderly. These studies attempt to estimate prevalence and incidence rates based on whether or not agencies have had

contact with cases of elder abuse or neglect, as well as to provide information about the causes of abuse. Descriptive data on abuse cases come from reports filled out by the respondents or direct interviews with agencies that report abuse cases. In essence, these surveys provide estimates about the extent to which different service professionals are familiar with elder abuse and neglect.

Based on these surveys, the range of professionals who have had contact with cases of elder abuse and neglect range from 55 percent (19) to nearly 100 percent (20,21). For example, in a recent survey of professionals, Dolan and Hendricks (22) mailed questionnaires to police officers and social service providers in two midwestern communities. Of the police officers reporting, 33 percent had encountered abuse or neglect; of the social service personnel reporting, 69 percent had encountered cases of elder abuse, sexual abuse, or neglect. This study, however, was designed more for exploring attitudes and practices of these groups in elder mistreatment than for assessing prevalence of elder abuse.

Two other studies used somewhat different designs from those noted above. Instead of gathering information directly from professionals, Lau and Kosberg (23) and Wolf, Godkin, and Pillemer (2) relied on agency case records. Lau and Kosberg reviewed records of patients at the Chronic Illness Center in Cleveland, Ohio. Of the 404 elderly clients served in a 12-month period, nearly 10 percent were identified as victims of mistreatment. Wolf et al. examined 39 cases of physical, psychological, or mental abuse by caseworkers at three model projects on elder abuse. The data abstracted from these cases were then used to develop a characterization of the victim and perpetrator of elder abuse. This study differed from Lau and Kosberg's research in that the researchers designed a data collection instrument based on the standardized assessment form used by the caseworkers. In both studies, however, researchers obtained data from professional accounts of maltreatment rather than from interviews with victims themselves.

Whereas all these studies provide descriptive data on elder abuse, professional reports about cases may not be completely reliable. Professionals may interpret the circumstances of each case in a radically different way from that of the individuals involved. The problem is further compounded by the fact that the abuse cases described by social service professionals are those that have come to the attention of agencies. Agency clients represent only a subsample of all victims. For example, Dolan and Hendricks (22) point out that because of perceived lack of effectiveness, police officers may be reluctant to offer a referral to certain agencies. Social service agencies may, therefore, see only a small percentage of the potential client population. Pillemer and Finkelhor's research (5) supports this notion; they estimate that fewer than 1 in 14 elder abuse cases are reported to agencies.

Case-control Studies

Several recent studies have attempted to go beyond previous efforts by (1) interviewing the victims themselves and (2) including a control group of nonabused elderly persons. One important issue in conducting case control studies is how the control group is determined, including the criteria used for matching cases and controls. For example, Phillips (3) and Hwalek, Sengstock, and Lawrence (24) conducted case-control studies in which the respondents were selected from social service agencies and assigned to abuse or nonabuse groups by service providers. Service providers who participated were asked to identify persons whom they believed were victims of abuse and neglect and to choose a nonabused control for each case.

Use of service professionals limits the outcomes in two ways. One is whether the information obtained discriminates between abused and non-abused elders or, instead, tells us about differences between persons whom professionals *identify* as abused and those they believe are not abused. Second, it is not clear what criteria, if any, are used for matching the cases and the controls.

Pillemer (25) conducted a study in which cases were identified from the caseloads of three model projects on elder abuse. These individuals were compared with a control group of elderly persons drawn from the non-abused caseload of one of the model projects. Furthermore, cases and controls were individually matched on sex and living arrangement. Similarly, Pillemer and Finkelhor (17) conducted a random sample survey of 1,911 elderly residents in the greater Boston area in which control cases were randomly selected from nonabused survey respondents. All the nonabused elders were asked about their relationship to a close relative to serve as a comparison to the relationship between the maltreated elderly and their abusers.

In a somewhat different case-control design, Bristowe and Collins (4) compared families in which appropriate care was delivered to elderly relatives and families where abusive caregiving situations existed. Profiles of the families were based on incident report forms completed by the service providers or reports received through media contacts. Control cases, however, were not matched with abusive cases. Instead, several control variables were used to ensure similarity of background characteristics of the groups, so that abuse was the principal distinguishing feature.

Interviewer bias is another issue in case-control studies. It is preferable to incorporate "blind" interviews into these studies in order to minimize the bias on the part of the interviewer. In the study conducted by Phillips (3), a blind interview technique was used in which interviewers were unaware whether the respondent was in the abused or nonabused group. In the Pillemer study (25), all interviews were conducted in person by the same interviewer. However, as in the study by Hwalek et al. (24) and Bristowe and Collins (4), the interviewer was aware of whether the respondent was an abuse or nonabuse case.

Finally, most case-control studies are weakened by their failure to distinguish among various kinds of maltreatment. To address this issue, Pillemer and Finkelhor (17) included three categories of maltreatment: physical abuse, neglect and chronic verbal aggression. Bristowe and Collins

(4) used four categories of maltreatment previously identified by Hickey and Douglass (26): passive neglect, active neglect, verbal abuse, and physical abuse.

Although the case-control studies reported here have several limitations, they clearly demonstrate the utility of more rigorous research designs. For example, some investigators have asserted that the abused elderly tend to be physically and/or mentally impaired. However, without a comparison group, it is impossible to know if abused elders are more or less impaired than other persons. In the next section on causal factors, it will become apparent that the findings of case-control studies contradict some previous assertions regarding the nature of elder abuse. It is only through the use of control groups that these observations were made possible.

Other Sources

Several secondary sources of data may provide important information about domestic violence against the elderly. In this section, we briefly discuss three sources: law enforcement agencies, health care providers, and state agencies.

Law Enforcement Agencies

One possible source of data is the Uniform Crime Reports (UCR) of the Federal Bureau of Investigation. For example, the UCR records the relationship between the assailant and victim in cases of homicide. One could investigate the cases in which parents or grandparents are murdered. Investigators should explore other possible analyses using UCR data. Other official sources of data on criminal behavior against the elderly include the police, the courts, and the prisons. Clearly, these records may be subject to underreporting, especially in the sensitive area of family violence. However, in the absence of other data, official crime statistics may shed valuable light on elder abuse.

Health Care Providers

Substantial amounts of data on child and wife abuse have been obtained from emergency rooms where the personnel are frequently the only service providers seen by victims of domestic violence. Victims often do not seek help unless their injuries are severe. Only recently have efforts been made to collect data on elder mistreatment cases from health providers. Specific reporting schemes for elder abuse cases have been developed for hospital personnel (27,28). In New York, the Victim Services Agency and Mt. Sinai Medical Center have joined together to address the problem of identifying and treating elder abuse victims. Through this project, data are being collected to determine the number and type of elder abuse cases and to understand the characteristics of persons involved in such family problems. As with crime statistics, such reports are subject to bias: only those cases in which abuse has resulted in serious injury are likely to be recorded.

State Agencies

By 1987 all states had established some form of system that records reports of elder abuse and neglect, with forty-three states having legislated mandatory reporting laws. Most states also have established special protective service agencies to intervene in elder abuse cases. In all these states, records are maintained on persons who are reported. Data from such reports compose a valuable source of data on abuse victims. In the mid-1980s the U.S. Administration on Aging funded a study in which information on reports of elder mistreatment was gathered from all 50 states. Tatara (29) used these data to estimate the national incidence of reports of elder abuse. Since statutes vary considerably among states, attempts to make national estimates are limited. Given these limitations, Tatara concluded that nationally, between 51,000 and 186,000 elderly persons were reported to the authorities as victims of some form of elder mistreatment in 1985. Such data have potential for contributing to the development of state and national policy in this area. More resources need to be made available to assemble state-level reports into data sets.

Data from all these sources are potentially very valuable. They do not, however, replace the need for the analytic studies discussed previously. The most pressing need is for random sample population surveys and rigorous case-control designs. Descriptive data can shed some light on the phenomenon of elder abuse, but inherent biases in such data limit their utility. The final section of this chapter suggests ways to improve research design.

RISK FACTORS

Characteristics of Abuse Victims

Despite their methodological limitations, previous studies suggest some fairly consistent findings regarding the abused elderly population. Most of the studies have found that the abused individuals tend to be female, although in Pillemer and Finkelhor's research (17), victims were evenly divided between men and women. Abused victims have also been generally found to be disproportionately "old-old" (75 and over). Many studies have found that victims experience increased vulnerability due to illness or impairment. Finally, it has been shown consistently that abused elders tend to live with the perpetrator of abuse. Unfortunately, these findings are the only ones that emerge reliably from the studies. Results relating to the frequency with which abuse occurs and the types of abuse most often found are virtually impossible to compare, because of the widely varying definitions employed. Further, few of the studies provide reliable evidence on the causes of elder abuse.

Causal Factors

A theoretical framework for understanding elder abuse cannot be derived from previous research on elder abuse. There are two areas of research, however, that are useful in approaching this issue. First, findings from the study of child and spouse abuse may shed light on elder abuse. However, although it is useful to consult the family violence literature, this should be done only with the knowledge that the elderly occupy a special status in our society. Any attempt to understand the dynamics of abuse situations must take into account theory and research relating specifically to the aged. We must ask: What is it that makes the elderly vulnerable to abuse? How does being old specifically pattern family violence? Second, we believe it is necessary to include the more general literature on relations between spouses, and between elderly and adult children. Findings related to the determinants of the quality of family relationships of the elderly can provide important insights into elder abuse, especially in concert with domestic violence literature.

The extensive research literature on these two topics is considered in the following discussion of the causal factors for elder abuse. It is only possible to outline in this selective review the most important issues that have emerged from the review:

1. Intraindividual dynamics (psychopathology of the abuser).
2. Intergenerational transmission of violent behavior ("cycle of violence").
3. Dependency and exchange relations between abuser and abused.
4. External stress.
5. Social isolation.

Intraindividual Dynamics*

Intra-individual theories emphasize pathological characteristics of the abuser as the primary cause of maltreatment. In previous studies, family researchers have found that psychological well-being is related to the general quality of family relationships. Various measures of psychological well-being have been consistently related to marital satisfaction both in the general population (30,31) and specifically among the elderly (32). Whereas the causal direction in these studies cannot be precisely determined, the psychological well-being of marriage partners clearly affects the quality of relationships.

Many early investigators of child abuse held that abusive parents suffered from some kind of psychological disease. Based on intraindividual perspectives, the cure for child abuse was to treat the emotional illness (33). Clinicians and practitioners tended to attribute abuse to sadistic personality traits (34), whereas other researchers traced abusive behavior to a flaw in the socialization process. Several investigators of wife abuse also traced such behavior to psychopathological traits in the abuser. Critics of the intraindividual explanations (33,35) have claimed that such investigations have lacked rigorous research methodologies and have failed to account for

---

*Material in this section is derived in large part from Wolf R, Pillemer K. Helping elderly victims: the reality of elder abuse (11).

structural factors, such as socioeconomic status, economic stress, and unemployment.

One intraindividual characteristic that has been emphasized by some investigators is the relationship between alcohol and drug abuse and family violence (36–38). Alcohol and drug consumption may diminish inhibitions against abusive acts or may instead provide an excuse for violent behavior carried out intentionally. Preliminary evidence has indicated that a similar relationship between substance abuse and domestic violence may exist among the elderly (2,39). Case-control studies are necessary to demonstrate a causal role for substance abuse in domestic violence against the elderly.

It should also be noted that the dynamics of elder abuse may differ from those of other forms of family violence. In particular, abusers of the elderly may be more likely to suffer from psychological problems than child or wife abusers. Some research has, in fact, provided evidence that persons who abuse the elderly are more likely to be developmentally disabled, mentally ill, or alcoholic (4,5,20,23,40).

Intergenerational Transmission of Violent Behavior
It has been become a widely held view that victims of child abuse grow up to be abusers. In fact, many researchers have postulated that children learn to be violent in family settings and use these learned behaviors when they become adults. This theory is sometimes summed up as a "cycle of violence." In one of the most extensive reviews of the spousal violence literature, Hotaling and Sugarman (41) found that the cumulative research evidence does indeed identify witnessing parental violence during childhood as one of the strongest risk factors for wife abuse as an adult. In a national survey, Straus, Gelles, and Steinmetz (14) found that the amount of physical punishment experienced as a child was positively associated with the rate of abusive violence to one's own children.

Whereas it is reasonable to postulate that abusers of the elderly will also be more likely to have been raised in violent families, at present, no evidence exists to support this hypothesis. It is important to note that a significant difference exists between elder abuse and other forms of domestic violence: in the case of elder abuse, the previous violence may be perpetuated, but the roles are reversed. The "cycle of violence" must therefore take an alternative form. Rather than becoming an abuser because one was abused by someone else, the cycle becomes much more direct: the formerly abused child strikes out against the abuser. This would appear to involve a different psychological process, one with elements of retaliation as well as imitation.

Dependency
Two competing theories have arisen that relate dependency to elder abuse. The first theory emphasizes the role of "caregiver stress" as a risk factor for maltreatment. Abuse is seen as resulting from the resentment generated by the increased dependency of an older, more impaired person on a caretaker. The second theory stresses the reverse configuration and suggests that the

increased dependency of the *abuser* on his or her victim leads to more maltreatment. These theories are discussed separately.

Concerning *caregiver stress*, the literature on family relations of the elderly supports the notion that dependency of an old person leads to poor-quality relationships with relatives. One of the most consistent findings is that parents' health is positively correlated with feelings of closeness and attachment between parents and their adult children (42–44). A likely reason for this pattern is the effect of declining parental health on the prior flow of support between the generations. As the parents' health declines, adult children may have to increase their support to the parent and possibly accept the cessation of assistance from the parent.

In fact, several studies have documented the negative effects of parental dependency. For example, Circirelli (45,46) found negative feelings on the part of adult children when both parental dependency and the amount of help needed from the child were high. Similarly, a study by Adams (47) revealed that affectional ties to widowed parents were weaker when adult children's help was not reciprocated. Thus it appears that when adult children feel the support relationship with a parent is inequitable, the quality of the relationship declines.

Many students of elder abuse have also emphasized the dependency of elderly persons on the abusive relative as a major cause of abuse (48–51). It is argued that families undergo stress when an elderly person becomes dependent on his or her relatives for care. Steinmetz and Amsden (48) suggested that families undergo "situational inversion" when the elderly person becomes dependent on his or her children for financial, physical, and/or emotional support, and this inversion leads to severe stress on the caregiver. As the costs of the relationship grow for the caregiver and the rewards diminish, the exchange becomes perceived as unfair. According to this view, caregivers who do not have the ability to escape or ameliorate the situation may become abusive.

This theory appears plausible, but there are few firm research findings to support it. It is clear from the gerontological literature that a substantial number of elderly persons are dependent on their spouses or other relatives (52–54). However, recent prevalence findings indicate that only a small minority (approximately 3%) of the elderly are abused (17). Since abuse occurs in only a small proportion of families, no direct correlation can be assumed between dependency of an older person and abuse. In fact, Phillips (3) failed to find any difference in level of impairment between a group of abused elderly and a control group, and Bristowe (55) found abused elders to be less impaired than a control group. Pillemer and Suitor (56) have shown that parents' health and dependency are not related to parent-child conflict when the generations share a residence.

Concerning *abuser dependency*, there is some evidence that a significant degree of dependency exists on the part of the abuser as well as the abused. Wolf, Strugnell, and Godkin (57) found a "web of mutual dependency" between abuser and abused. In two-thirds of their cases, the perpetrator was reported to be financially dependent on the victim. Hwalek et al. (24), in a case-control study, also found that the financial dependency of the abuser on the elderly victim was an important risk factor in elder abuse. A study based on interviews with abusers of the elderly also supports the hypothesis that the dependency of relatives, rather than the elder, is an important risk factor for abuse (40).

Pillemer's (39) and Pillemer and Finkelhor's (5) results support this argument even more strongly. Their research found that abusers in the sample were much more likely to be dependent on their victims financially and in a variety of other areas. In general, abusers were found to be heavily dependent individuals, including disabled or cognitively impaired spouses and children.

This finding that the continued dependence of an adult child or spouse upon an elderly victim is related to physical violence may seem counterintuitive. A theoretical explanation of the phenomenon can be derived from social exchange theory and the concept of power. Finkelhor (58), in his attempt to identify common features of family abuse, noted that abuse can occur as a response to a perceived powerlessness. It may be that the feeling of powerlessness experienced by an adult child who is still dependent on an elderly parent is especially acute because it violates society's expectations for normal adult behavior.

In summary, the role of dependency deserves serious attention. However, it is not clear yet who is depending on whom in these abusive relationships. Perhaps a better way to conceptualize the issue is to view a serious imbalance of dependency in either direction as a potential risk factor. Researchers must explore the role of both types of inequity in elder abuse. In order to shed light on the issue of dependency, such factors as the need for assistance of the abused, feelings of caregiving burden on the part of the abuser, and the dependency of the abuser must be examined.

External Stress

A number of investigators have found a positive relationship between external stress (as differentiated from the stress that results from interpersonal relationships in the family) and child and wife abuse (14,59,60). In contrast to the intra-individual and social psychological explanations of risk factors for elder abuse, this perspective provides a sociocultural explanation. Accordingly, this perspective emphasizes social-structural, macro-level variables such as unemployment and economic conditions. However, the social stress model alone cannot explain elder abuse, as it does not explain why some families respond to stress with abuse and others do not. To date, no systematic exploration has been conducted of the relationship between stress and elder abuse, although Sengstock and Liang (61) and Pillemer and Finkelhor (17) provide some preliminary evidence that such a relationship exists. Based on the strength of findings relating stress to other forms of family violence, this area would also appear to be an important one for future investigators.

Social Isolation

Social isolation has also been found to be characteristic of families in which other forms of domestic violence occurs (59,60,62,63). This is probably because behaviors that are considered illegitimate tend to be hidden. Detection of abusive actions can result in informal sanctions from friends, kin, and neighbors, and formal sanctions from police and the courts. Thus, all forms of family violence are likely to be less frequent in families that have friends or relatives who live nearby (64). The presence of an active social network may be a particularly strong deterrent to elder abuse because the abuse is viewed as a highly illegitimate behavior. In two separate case-control studies, Phillips (3) and Pillemer (25) found abused elderly persons more likely to be socially isolated than nonabused persons.

In summary, the literature points to five major risk factors that could lead to elder abuse: intraindividual dynamics, intergenerational transmission of violent behavior, dependency, external stress, and isolation. In the framework proposed here, these factors may directly precipitate elder maltreatment. To the extent that a family has one or more of these characteristics, it may be at a greater risk of elder abuse. Further, it was noted that the risk of elder abuse may be higher for persons who share a residence with others, and who are married.

OUTCOMES

Little is known about the consequences of elder abuse. In what is probably the most comprehensive literature review to date, Hudson and Johnson (7) do not cite any evidence relating to the impact of abuse on victims. Some data do exist, however, on physical manifestations or descriptions of physical injuries, such as bruises and sprains, abrasions, bone fractures, burns, and wounds (2,15,19,61). Anecdotal evidence suggests that victimization does produce negative psychological outcomes, although sound empirical findings are scarce.

Evidence from child-abuse and wife-abuse literature indicates that victims suffer negative psychological consequences. Physically abused children have been found to have lower self-esteem and to be less effective in interaction with peers, more likely to inappropriately interpret other's behaviors, more aggressive, and more likely to have an external locus of control than nonabused children (65).

A limited amount of literature also exists on psychological outcomes of wife abuse. Blackman (66) describes a process of psychological changes in which the victim eventually enters a "learned helplessness" phase and then focuses energy into survival. Browne (67) also notes a variety of long-term consequences of wife abuse, including confusion and feelings of powerlessness and helplessness, increased dependency on others, depression, disturbed eating and sleeping patterns, and a sense of isolation.

The question then arises whether similar outcomes have been observed in elder abuse victims. Certainly, clinical and case study data have documented that some elders experience severe emotional distress as a consequence of maltreatment (2,50). Phillips (3), the only investigator to have examined this issue using a case-control design, found victims of elder abuse and neglect to be significantly more likely to be depressed. Using data from a random sample survey of elder abuse and neglect, Pillemer and Prescott (65) examined psychological consequences of abuse victimization. The investigators found that persons who were maltreated reported higher levels of depression, even when controlling for health, age, gender, and marital status. In conjunction with the study by Phillips (3), it seems clear that abused elderly are significantly more likely to be depressed than nonvictims. However, it is not clear whether depression is an antecedent or consequence of maltreatment. Further research should be conducted that involves direct interviews with victims as well as longitudinal studies.

The documentation of the physical consequences of maltreatment is equally difficult to achieve. Such effects may be confounded with the normal physical changes that accompany aging and/or various physical impairments. As previously stated, it would be difficult to determine which physical indicator is an antecedent or a consequence of maltreatment. The concern about the long-term consequences of mistreatment, however, has important policy implications. For instance, abuse victims may use health care services and depend on support services more than nonabused elderly.

Researchers should begin to take into account the range of possible consequences of elder abuse and to collect data on the incidence and nature of such outcomes. Such information is vital to efforts to formulate and support interventions in elder abuse situations.

INTERVENTIONS

It has been over ten years since the problem of elder abuse and neglect first came to the public's attention. However, our ability to design meaningful prevention and intervention strategies and programs is greatly handicapped by our lack of knowledge regarding the extent, nature, and dynamics of elder abuse. In the absence of a comprehensive national policy regarding maltreatment of the elderly, states and communities have designed their own programs to help abused persons and their families. A wide variety of services has been initiated, ranging from elder protective services to family counseling to legal intervention. The different intervention strategies adopted thus far by practitioners and policymakers can be placed into three basic categories: mandatory reporting laws, protective services programs, and direct services. Of these intervention strategies, mandatory reporting and protective services have become the favored responses to elder abuse; both are highly controversial. At present, one of the greatest gaps in information about elder maltreatment is the lack of evaluation data regarding various types of interventions. We briefly review these two initiatives and then discuss service options for abuse victims and their families.

Mandatory Reporting Laws

All 50 states now have mandatory reporting laws that cover the elderly in some ways. Mandatory reporting laws require certain groups of people to report suspected cases of abuse to designated authorities. The goal of these laws is to identify abused older people and thereby allow the state to intervene in their situations. There is, however, tremendous variation from state to state in the laws. Definitions vary as to who should be classified as abused. The agencies authorized to receive reports are most often state welfare or social service departments, and less frequently law enforcement agencies, local social service agencies, and state units on aging. Usually, the agency designated to receive reports has the responsibility for investigation.

Elder abuse legislation is not without controversy. Proponents of mandatory reporting argue that such laws are the best method for bringing cases to light. They hold that without these statutes, few persons would report cases of suspected abuse.

In contrast, opponents have cited several reasons for not recommending mandatory reporting laws. First, critics claim that there is no evidence yet that mandatory reporting is effective (68–70). One early study (71) concluded that the increase in the number of reports filed with the authorized agencies was more likely a result of the increase in publicity about the problem of elder abuse (including the passage of legislation) than the mandatory provision of the laws. Further, penalties for not reporting are rarely, if ever, enforced.

Second, some critics have noted that states feel they have done their job after the law is passed and have failed to provide sufficient funds for services to victims and abusers (68). In such cases, a small staff must attempt to handle the large number of referrals that come in response to the law.

Third, many claim that the reporting process interferes with the relationship and confidentiality between professionals and clients. This presents these professionals with a dilemma: either to violate the law or break trust of a client and possibly jeopardize a therapeutic relationship.

Finally, critics of mandatory elder abuse reporting believe that in using the child abuse model, proponents are adopting a set of assumptions that are not applicable to older people. The implications drawn from the analogy to child abuse are that elders are incompetent and unable to report themselves. Such inferences infantilize the elder's position in society, foster negative stereotypes of the aged, and limit older persons' ability to control their own lives (72, p. 731).

In their evaluation of an elder abuse intervention project, Wolf and Pillemer (11) found that mandatory reporting did not necessarily lead to a greater number of reports of elder abuse, but did lead to a high number of referrals, all of which had to be investigated. Because the number of staff necessary to carry out all the investigations was often greater than the agency was able to provide, staff were unable to focus on the most serious cases, and this led to worker frustration.

Thus a major controversy exists over mandatory reporting. Caution is urged in regarding this type of legislation as an appropriate response to elder abuse. Mandatory reporting statutes *must* be carefully evaluated to determine their effectiveness. At a minimum, mandatory reporting must be accompanied by a substantial commitment of resources to the designated reporting agency.

Protective Services

Protective services programs for the elderly are equally controversial. Most public protective services programs assign a legal intervention role to social workers who investigate cases of abuse and attempt to treat the situation, bringing services where needed. Such programs generally also involve the use of legal surrogate options, such as guardianship or conservatorship, when the elderly person is judged to be incompetent (73, p. 3).

There have been numerous critics of protective services for the elderly. The strongest critics have been members of the legal community. They see such programs as an intrusion upon the civil liberties of the elderly and as a way of infantilizing them. They argue that most states define abuse too broadly, and that they allow for a potentially stigmatizing intrusion into families with merely the normal range of human problems (74). Further, critics hold that guardianship, which takes away many of the rights of an old person, is frequently used when it is not warranted.

In order to be effective, protective service programs need a strategy that reduces the tension within the legal community and alleviates the ambiguity and multiplicity of tasks performed by the protective service agencies. Bergman (75) and Bergeron (76) suggest a systematic or holistic approach in which protective services can be more effective in handling long-term problems, instead of providing quick-fix solutions (75, p. 96). Bergman suggests a systematic combination of specific crisis intervention and protective services strategies, whereas Bergeron calls for the integration of adult protective services system with human service providers.

Service Options

Communities have initiated a wide range of service programs for abused elderly. These service options tend to be based on one of two assumptions. The first assumption is that the dependency of the victim causes maltreatment. Based on this assumption, most discussions of service needs of abused elders list health and social services that are not specific to abuse. Such services are generally most appropriate for cases in which the victim is old, functionally impaired, and dependent, and in which the abuse is related to strain on the caregivers. In many cases, an attempt is made to introduce home care services, such as housekeeping and meal preparation, to relieve the burden of caregiving. Although such services may play a role in preventing or ameliorating abuse situations, research evidence indicates that this pattern of elderly abuse occurs in only a minority of cases.

In other cases, the victim is a relatively independent person who is abused by a dependent relative. Service options based on this second assumption require a different set of interventions. It has been argued that cases of elder abuse have close parallels with the situation of abused spouses, that is, they often involve legally independent adults who share a residence out of choice for a variety of material and emotional reasons. Several interventions that have been effective with victims of wife abuse may therefore benefit abused elders.

One such option is to increase social support for the elderly. For example, the battered women's movement, as noted earlier, has made much use of self-help groups. One important component of such groups has been consciousness-raising. Battered women and their advocates have gone to great lengths to convey to group members that they have a right to be free from violence, and that its use cannot be justified.

Another service option is the use of "safe houses" or emergency shelters by elderly victims. Battered women's advocates have relied heavily on such locations to protect abused victims. This model presumes that after escaping from the abuse, the victim can either begin to live independently or can return to the abuser who becomes aware that she will no longer tolerate abuse. Often cited as a much-needed resource for helping elderly victims, emergency shelters of various types and forms are being developed in communities both here and abroad.

A final alternative is legal action. The parallel to spouse abuse suggests that criminal justice sanctions could be more widely used in cases of elderly abuse. Sherman and Berk (77) have provided important evidence that police intervention may reduce further episodes of wife abuse. In one experiment, they found that arrest was the most effective method to prevent further episodes of wife abuse. There are other ways in which the police can become involved as well. They are often the first people on the scene in response to a complaint of elder abuse. Consequently, they are in a unique position to link victims with effective community services.

Police departments are only one of many types of community agencies that are becoming concerned with the problem of elder abuse and neglect. Many communities have created task forces of service providers and other interested individuals who attempt to raise the consciousness of professionals and lay people regarding the needs of abused and neglected elders.

The above examples represent exciting steps in the effort to prevent and treat elder abuse and neglect. Based on observations of intervention projects, Wolf and Pillemer (11) and Hwalek, Hill, and Stahl (78) suggest that the real solution to elder abuse and neglect lies in the development of a comprehensive service system to meet the needs of victims and their families.

Recommendations

Rather than merely summarizing the information we have presented in earlier sections of this chapter, we will conclude with a set of recommendations for improving knowledge of elder abuse. Given the lack of firm research, we believe that it is more appropriate to make proposals for future research rather than directly for practice and policy. The most critical need at present appears to be for information about the incidence and causes of elder abuse; without this, plans for intervention into the problem of elder abuse are, at best, educated guesses, and at worst, opportunistic political compromises. It should be noted that most of these recommendations are applicable to other forms of maltreatment besides physical abuse (e.g., psychological abuse, material abuse, and neglect).

1. Investigators should design studies based on direct interviews with abused elders. Victims will talk, and often at great length, about the maltreatment. This is evidenced by the work of Bristowe and Collins (4), Phillips (3), Pillemer (25), and others. Failing to interview victims in investigations on elder abuse can no longer be justified. Whereas assessment data compiled by competent professionals may accurately describe certain aspects of the case, understanding of the family dynamics that produced maltreatment ultimately relies on direct interviews with the parties involved.

2. Future studies must move away from agency samples towards general population surveys. The results of Pillemer and Finkelhor's prevalence survey (17) of one metropolitan area show that agency caseloads are not necessarily representative of the types or numbers of cases in the population. A national incidence survey is greatly needed to learn the magnitude of the problem and to provide a more complete picture of conflict and violence. Further, a national voluntary reporting system with standards accepted by states for reporting cases is needed to provide a national profile of reported cases.

3. The importance of control group designs cannot be overemphasized. It is only through this methodology that certain characteristics of the victims are identified. For instance, the findings that physically abused elders are often less impaired than nonabused elders, and that perpetrators are more dependent than caregivers of nonabused persons, were only obtainable through case-control studies.

4. Researchers in this field should study abusers. A study based on interviews with perpetrators has been conducted by Anetzberger (40). Based on her typology of abuse perpetrators, Anetzberger recommends a need to differentiate intervention strategies by the configuration of abuser characteristics (79, p. 50). Although her small sample size calls into question the generalizability of the results, the suggestive findings point out the need for more studies in this area.

5. Research in this field should begin to focus to a greater degree on the consequences of abuse. What effects does being an elder abuse victim have on an individual? "Learned helplessness" has been shown to result from wife

abuse (80). Does this also hold for abused elders? Do abused elders suffer decrements in psychological well-being? What are the consequences of maltreatment in terms of service needs and utilization by abused victims? This area holds promise for future research.

6. Investigators should pay more attention to the context of abusive acts. Does an argument precede abuse? Have one or both persons usually been drinking prior to the incident? Are others generally present? More specifics regarding the circumstances in which domestic violence against the elderly occur are necessary.

7. Existing intervention programs should be systematically evaluated. At present we know very little regarding the effectiveness of various types of intervention into elder abuse cases. Little research has been conducted on whether programs currently in operation benefit those they serve, or whether they may in fact have negative effects on clients. A number of demonstration programs have been initiated to test the efficacy of alternative models of delivering health services to older adults. Evaluation of current projects is needed to assist in creating new intervention programs or in redesigning current projects. Two recent evaluation projects have provided several recommendations regarding the organization and delivery of services. In Illinois, Hwalek et al. (78) evaluated four state-funded elder abuse demonstration projects. The outcome of their evaluation was then used to design a statewide plan for managing elder abuse cases. Based on an evaluation of three Model Projects on Elder Abuse in New England, Wolf and Pillemer (11) suggest that community-based programs in conjunction with interagency coordination are important contributors to successful intervention.

A high priority for researchers must be to use sophisticated evaluation research techniques to determine the impact of treatment programs. Without such careful evaluation, funds may be wasted on inappropriate services that fail to help—and may even harm—elder abuse victims and their families.

ACKNOWLEDGMENTS

We are grateful to Karen E. Hayden, Research Assistant, Family Research Laboratory for her contributions to this chapter.

ANNOTATED BIBLIOGRAPHY

Breckman RS, Adelman RD. Strategies for helping victims of elder mistreatment. Beverly Hills, CA: Sage, 1988.

This book provides a practical guide for students, physicians, social service and health workers, and professionals in dealing with the difficult social problem of elder abuse and neglect. In chapters one and two, a theoretical framework for understanding elder mistreatment is presented. Subsequent chapters explore various aspects of the overall topic, such as the relationship between gerontological and family violence knowledge and elder mistreatment, a review of the signs and symptoms of mistreatment, a framework for assessing mistreatment, and intervention strategies. Appendices include clinical materials for use by professionals working with victims of elder mistreatment. The authors conclude with suggestions for future directions in the areas of research, training, and program development.

Callahan JJ Jr. Elder abuse: Some questions for policy makers. Gerontologist 1989; 28:453–458.

A critical perspective on elder abuse as a social problem is offered and the difficulty in developing programs to address an issue that has yet to be "universally defined" is discussed. The author suggests a "broad social service approach" that meets the varied needs of all older persons, rather than a redistribution of funds within the entire social service system already in need of resources. He also finds that the already enacted criminal laws on elder abuse should be enforced, and that more information about the needs of all older persons be made available to professionals, caretakers, and older people themselves. The author suggests further research on the outcomes of social interventions of family violence, and stresses the need to provide older persons with the "economic means for a decent life and the opportunity to exercise their own choices."

Filinson R, Ingman S. Elder abuse: Practice and policy. New York: Human Services Press, 1989.

The authors provide an overview of programs and policies developed in response to the original research findings on elder abuse. Section I presents a critical examination of the early research findings that were crucial for the formulation of various policy initiatives. Section II focuses on the obstacles encountered by different practitioners in the recognition and assessment of elder abuse. Section III addresses policy developments and consequences on the federal, state, and local levels. The goal of this book is to encourage reconsideration of responses to elder abuse given accumulating evidence from various intervention strategies and better designed research.

Kosberg JI, ed. Abuse and maltreatment of the elderly: Causes and interventions. Boston: John Wright, PSG, Inc., 1983.

This book provides an overview of causes and consequences of victimization and possible interventions by those committed to working with the elderly. Section I deals with problems faced by the elderly, including crime, maltreatment within institutional settings, elder abuse within the family, exploitation, and ageism. Section II focuses on groups of elderly especially vulnerable to victimization, including aged black Americans, the disabled, elderly women, the aged in public housing or urban areas, and elderly parents. Section III discusses intervention possibilities such as individual and family treatment, community organization and advocacy efforts, legal and health professional activities, state and local programs, and national legislation.

Phillips LR. Abuse and neglect of the frail elderly at home: An exploration of theoretical relationships. J Nursing 1983; 8:379–392.

The study reported in this article employed a purposive sample of 74 elderly persons who were identified as either having a "good relationship" or an "abusive/neglectful relationship" to their caregivers. This data showed that demographic characteristics and variables like anger, hostility, stress, and level of impairment were similar between the two groups. Significant differences included lower expectations of the abused subjects for their caregivers and more depression in the abuse group.

Pillemer K. The dangers of dependency: New findings on domestic violence against the elderly. Social Problems 1985; 33:146–158.

In this article, the author examines conflicting hypotheses that (1) increased dependency of an older person causes stress for relatives who then respond with physical violence, versus (2) increased dependency of the abusive relative leads to maltreatment.

Both qualitative and quantitative analyses of this case-control study indicate that the elderly victims were not more dependent, but rather they were more likely to be supporting their dependent abuser. The author stresses that future research and policy attention focus on the perpetrator of abuse.

Pillemer K, Finkelhor D. The prevalence of elder abuse: A random sample survey. Gerontologist 1988; 28:51–57.

The authors present the first large-scale stratified random sample survey of elder abuse and neglect. Two-stage interviews were conducted on 2,020 community-dwelling persons of 65 years or older in the greater Boston area. The study focuses on three forms of mistreatment: physical abuse, psychological abuse, and neglect. The researchers found a prevalence rate of 32 abused elderly per 1,000 population, the largest proportion of which is spouse abuse. The authors outline the characteristics of victims and suggest implications for policy and practice. Implications include: service providers to the elderly be educated about abuse, specifically spouse abuse; the elderly themselves be educated on spouse abuse; and services be tailored to the problem of spouse abuse among the elderly population.

Wolf RS, Anderson SM, eds. J Elder Abuse and Neglect, vol. 1, 1989. Redding, CA: Hawthorne Press.

Designated the official publication of the National Committee for Prevention of Elder Abuse, the objective of the journal is to act as a "forum for the discussion of scientific investigations, program developments, policy initiatives, and personal commentary about the maltreatment of elderly and disabled persons." Its major goal is to play a significant part in the education of professionals and the public concerning the problem of elder abuse. The first issue includes articles that addresses basic theoretical, empirical, and practical issues of mistreatment from the perspectives of academicians and clinicians.

Wolf RS, Pillemer KA. Helping elderly victims. New York: Columbia University Press, 1989.

This book presents findings from a three-year study of three Administration on Aging Model Projects on Elder Abuse and Neglect. Discussion includes a review of previous research and expected theories of causation, the factors related to the types of abuse and neglect, model performance, and outcome. Implications for practice, program development, and policy are given as well as some hypotheses concerning the dynamics of the abusive situation.

REFERENCES

1. Pedrick-Cornell C, Gelles RJ. Elder abuse: The status of current knowledge. Family Relations 1982; 31:457–465.
2. Wolf R, Godkin MA, Pillemer K. Elder abuse and neglect: Report from three model projects. Worcester: University of Massachusetts Medical Center, 1984.
3. Phillips LR. Abuse and neglect of the frail elderly at home: An exploration of theoretical relationships. J Advanced Nursing 1983; 8:379–392.
4. Bristowe E, Collins JB. Family mediated abuse of noninstitutionalized frail elderly men and women living in British Columbia. J Elder Abuse Neglect 1989; 1:45–64.
5. Pillemer K, Finkelhor D. Causes of elder abuse: Caregiver stress versus problem relatives. Am J Orthopsychiatry 1989; 59:179–187.
6. Hudson M. Analysis of the concepts of elder maltreatment: Abuse and neglect. J Elder Abuse Neglect 1989; 1:5–25.

7. Hudson M, Johnson T. Elder abuse and neglect: A review of the literature. In: Eisdorfer C, ed. Annual review of gerontology. New York: Springer, 1987.
8. Fulmer T, Ashley J. Neglect: What part of abuse? Pride Institute Journal of Long-Term Health Care 1986; 5:18–24.
9. Hudson M. Elder mistreatment: Current research. In: Pillemer K, Wolf R, eds. Elder abuse: Conflict in the family. Dover, MA: Auburn House, 1986: 125–166.
10. Yin P. Victimization of the aged. Springfield, IL: Charles C Thomas, 1985.
11. Wolf RS, Pillemer KA. Helping elderly victims: The reality of elder abuse. New York: Columbia University Press, 1989.
12. Johnson T. Critical issues in the definition of elder maltreatment. In: Elder abuse: Conflict in the family. Dover, MA: Auburn House, 1986: 167–195.
13. Breckman R, Adelman R. Strategies for helping victims of elder maltreatment. Beverly Hills, CA: Sage, 1988.
14. Straus M, Gelles RJ, Steinmetz S. Behind closed doors: Violence in the American family. New York: Doubleday, 1980.
15. Block MR, Sinnott JD. Battered elder syndrome: An exploratory study. College Park: University of Maryland, Center on Aging, 1979.
16. Gioglio RG, Blakemore P. Elder abuse in New Jersey: The knowledge and experience of abuse among older New Jerseyans. Trenton: NJ Dept. of Human Services, 1983.
17. Pillemer K, Finkelhor D. Prevalence of elder abuse: A random sample survey. Gerontologist 1988; 28:51–57.
18. Podnieks E, Pillemer K. Final report on survey of elder abuse in Canada. Ottawa, Ontario: Health and Welfare, Canada, 1989.
19. O'Malley T, O'Malley HC, Perez R, Mitchell V, Knuepfel GM. Elder abuse in Massachusetts: A survey of professionals and paraprofessionals. Boston: Legal Research and Services for the Elderly, 1979.
20. Douglas RL, Hickey T, Noel C. A study of maltreatment of the elderly and other vulnerable adults. Ann Arbor: University of Michigan, Institute of Gerontology, 1980.
21. Chen PN, Bell SL, Dolinsky DL, Doyle J, Dunn M. Elder abuse in domestic settings: A pilot study. J Gerontological Social Work 1981; 4:3–17.
22. Dolan R, Hendricks J. An exploratory study comparing attitudes and practices of police officers and social service providers in elder abuse and neglect cases. J Elder Abuse Neglect 1989; 1:75–90.
23. Lau E, Kosberg J. Abuse of the elderly by informal care providers. Aging Sept./Oct. 1979: 10–15.
24. Hwalek M, Sengstock M, Lawrence R. Assessing the probability of abuse of the elderly. Presentation at the Annual Meeting of the Gerontological Society of America, San Francisco, November 1984.
25. Pillemer K. Risk factors in elder abuse: Results from a case-control study. In: Pillemer K, Wolf RS, eds. Elder abuse: Conflict in the family. Dover, MA: Auburn House, 1986: 239–263.
26. Hickey T, Douglass R. Neglect and abuse of older family members: Professionals' perspectives and case experiences. Gerontologist 1981; 21:171–176.
27. Fulmer T, Cahill V. Assessing elder abuse: A study. J Gerontological Nursing 1984; 10:16–20.
28. O'Malley T, Everitt D, O'Malley H. Identifying and preventing family-mediated abuse and neglect of elderly persons. Ann Intern Med 1983; 98:998–1005.
29. Tatara T. Toward the development of estimates of national incidence of reports

of elder abuse based on currently available state data: An exploratory study. In: Filinson R, Ingman S, eds. Elder abuse: Practice and policy. New York: Human Services Press, 1989: 153–165.

30. Andrews FM, Withy SB. Social indicators of well-being: Americans' perceptions of life quality. New York: Plenum, 1979.

31. Glenn N, Weaver C. A multivariate, multisurvey study of marital happiness. J Marriage Family 1981; 40:269–282.

32. Lee G. Marriage and morale in later life. J Marriage Family 1978; 40:131–139.

33. Gelles RJ. Child abuse as psychopathology: A sociological critique and reformulation. In: Steinmetz S, Straus, MA, eds. Violence in the family. New York: Dodd, Mead, 1974: 190–204.

34. Young L. In: Steinmetz S, Straus MA, eds. Violence in the family. New York: Dodd, 1974: 187–189.

35. Gelles RJ, Straus MA. How violent are American families: Estimates from the National Family Violence Survey and other studies. In: Hotaling G et al. New directions in family violence research. Beverly Hills, CA: Sage, 1989.

36. Kantor G, Straus M. Substance abuse as a precipitant of family violence victimization. Presentation at the American Criminology Meeting, Atlanta, 1986.

37. Coleman D, Straus MA. Alcohol abuse and family violence. Durham, NH: University of New Hampshire, Family Violence Research Program, 1981.

38. Sedge S. Spouse abuse. In: Block M, Sinnott J, eds. The battered elder syndrome. College Park: University of Maryland, Center on Aging, 1979: 33–48.

39. Pillemer K. The dangers of dependency: New findings on domestic violence against the elderly. Social Problems 1985; 33:146–158.

40. Anetzberger GJ. Etiology of elder abuse by adult offspring. Springfield, IL: Charles C Thomas, 1987.

41. Hotaling G, Sugarman D. An analysis of risk markers in husband to wife violence: The current state of knowledge. Violence and Victims 1986; 1:101–124.

42. Baruch G, Barnett RC. Adult daughters' relationships with their mothers. J Marriage Family 1983; 45:601–606.

43. Cicirelli VG. Helping elderly parents: The role of adult children. Boston: Auburn House, 1981.

44. Johnson ES, Bursk BJ. Relationships between the elderly and their adult children. Gerontologist 1977; 17:90–96.

45. Cicirelli VG. Adult children and their parents. In: Brubaker TH, ed. Family relations in later life. Beverly Hills, CA: Sage, 1983.

46. Cicirelli VG. Adult children's attachment and helping behavior to elderly parents: A path model. J Marriage Family 1983; 45:815–825.

47. Adams BN. Kinship in an urban setting. Chicago: Markham, 1968.

48. Steinmetz SK, Amsden DJ. Dependency, family stress, and abuse. In: Brubaker TH, ed. Family relationships in later life. Beverly Hills, CA: Sage, 1983: 173–192.

49. Steinmetz SK. Dependency, stress and violence between middle-aged caregivers and their elderly parents. In: Kosberg JI, ed. Abuse and maltreatment of the elderly. Littleton, MA: John Wright PGS, 1983.

50. Quinn MJ, Tomita S. Elder abuse and neglect: Causes, diagnosis, and intervention strategies. New York: Springer, 1986.

51. Davidson JL. Elder abuse. In: Block MR, Sinnott JD, eds. Battered elder syndrome: An exploratory study. College Park: University of Maryland, Center on Aging, 1979.

52. Brody EM. Informal support system and health of the future aged. In: Gaitz CM, ed. Aging 2000: Our health care destiny. Vol. 2: Pyschological and policy issues. New York: Springer, 1985.

53. Cantor MH. Strain among caregivers: A study of experience in the United States. Gerontologist 1983; 23:597-604.

54. Kulys R, Tobin S. Older people and their "responsible others." Social Work 1980; 25:138-145.

55. Bristowe E, Collins JB. Family mediated abuse of noninstitutionalized frail elderly men and women living in British Columbia. J Elder Abuse Neglect 1989; 1:45-64.

56. Pillemer K, Suitor JJ. Elder abuse. In: Van Hasselt V, et al., eds. Handbook of family violence. New York: Plenum, 1988.

57. Wolf R, Strugnell C, Godkin M. Preliminary findings from the three model projects on elder abuse. Worcester: University of Massachusetts Medical Center, 1982.

58. Finkelhor D. Common features of family abuse. In: Finkelhor D, Gelles RJ, Hotaling G, Straus M, eds. Dark side of families: Current family violence research. Beverly Hills, CA: Sage, 1983: 17-26.

59. Gil DG. Violence against children: Physical abuse in the United States. Cambridge, MA: Harvard University Press, 1971.

60. Justice B, Justice R. The abusing family. New York: Human Services Press, 1976.

61. Sengstock MC, Laing J. Identifying and characterizing elder abuse. Detroit: Wayne State Institute of Gerontology, 1982.

62. Gelles RJ. The violent home. Beverly Hills, CA: Sage, 1972.

63. Stark E, Flitcraft A, Zuckerman D, Gray A, Robinson J, Frazier W. Wife abuse in the medical setting: An introduction to health personnel. Washington, DC: National Clearinghouse on Domestic Violence, 1981.

64. Nye FI. Choice, exchange and the family. In: Burr WR, Hill R, Nye FI, Reiss IL. Contemporary theories about the family. New York: Free Press, 1979: 1-14.

65. Pillemer K, Prescott D. Psychological effects of elder abuse: A research note. J Elder Abuse Neglect 1989; 1:65-72.

66. Blackman J. A narrowed vision: Clarity and clouds in victims of family violence. Presentation at the Third National Conference for Family Violence Researchers, Durham, NH, July 1987.

67. Browne A. When battered women kill. New York: Free Press, 1986.

68. Crystal S. Social policy and elder abuse. In: Pillemer KA, Wolf RS, eds. Elder abuse: Conflict in the family. Dover, MA: Auburn House, 1986: 331-339.

69. Faulkner LR. Mandating the reporting of suspected cases of elder abuse: An inappropriate, ineffective and ageist response to the abuse of older adults. Family Law Quarterly 1982; 16:69-91.

70. Callahan JJ. Elder abuse programming: Will it help the elderly? Urban Social Change Rev 1982; 15:15-19.

71. Alliance Elder Abuse Project. An analysis of state's mandatory reporting laws on elder abuse. Syracuse, NY: Alliance/Catholic Charities, 1981.

72. Lee D. Mandatory reporting of elder abuse: A cheap but ineffective solution to the problem. Fordham Urban Law J 1986; 14:131-139.

73. Callendar W. Improving protective services for older Americans: A national guide series. Portland: Center for Research and Advanced Study, University of Southern Maine, 1982.

74. Callahan JJ. Elder abuse programming: Will it help the elderly? Presentation at the National Conference on the Abuse of Older Persons, Boston, 1981.

75. Bergman JA. Responding to abuse and neglect cases: Protective services versus crisis intervention. In: Filinson R, Ingman S, eds. Elder abuse: Practice and policy. New York: Human Services Press, 1989: 94–103.

76. Bergeron LR. Elder abuse prevention: A holistic approach. In: Filinson R, Ingman S, eds. Elder abuse: Practice and policy. New York: Human Services Press, 1989: 218–228.

77. Sherman LW, Berk RA. Minneapolis domestic violence experiment. Police Foundation Reports, vol. 1, April 1984.

78. Hwalek M, Hill B, Stahl C. Illinois plan for a statewide abuse program. In: Filinson R, Ingson S, eds. Elder abuse: Practice and policy. New York: Human Services Press, 1989: 196–207.

79. Anetzberger GJ. Implications of research on elder abuse perpetrators: Rethinking current social policy and programming. In: Filinson R, Ingman S, eds. Elder abuse: Practice and policy. New York: Human Services Press, 1989: 43–50.

80. Walker L. Battered women and learned helplessness. Victimology 1977–1978; 2:535–534.

8

Suicide

PATRICK W. O'CARROLL, MARK L. ROSENBERG,
AND JAMES A. MERCY

As the eighth leading cause of death in the United States, suicide accounted for 30,796 deaths in 1987. Although the highest rates still occur among the elderly, the ranking of suicide as the fifth leading cause of premature death reflects an increasing incidence of suicide among adolescents and young adults. Men of all age and race groups are more likely than women to commit suicide, and white men are at highest risk.

Firearms are the most frequently used method of suicide for both men and women; from 1970 to 1984, the proportion of suicides committed with firearms increased 17 percent for men and 59 percent for women. The second method of choice for men is by hanging, and the third, poisoning by gas. The second choice for women is ingestion of an overdose of drugs.

The epidemiologic information concerning attempted suicide is meager and there is no uniformly accepted definition of suicide attempt. In one large multisite survey of U.S. adults, approximately three out of every 1,000 reported that they had "attempted suicide in the preceding year." The results of this survey (8) parallel other smaller surveys and suggest that there are approximately 25 suicide attempts for every completed suicide and that there are 750,000 adults who attempt suicide each year.

Data on suicide mortality are derived from death certificates. As a cause of death, suicide has been succinctly defined as death from intentionally self-inflicted injury. Yet applying this definition can be very difficult because determination of intention may require a retrospective collection of information regarding the decedent's state of mind prior to death. The quality and amount of this information as well as the ability of the official who is responsible for the certification varies greatly from case to case. In addition, the social stigma associated with suicide may make some coroners and medical examiners reluctant to certify suicide as the cause of death. Because of these limitations, it is highly likely that official suicide statistics substantially underestimate the true suicide rate. There are no national data sources for the magnitude of the physical and mental health consequences of attempted suicide or for the incidence of attempted suicide among persons under 18 years of age.

Risk factors for suicide include certain psychiatric illnesses, personality disorders (particularly borderline and antisocial personality disorders), alcoholism, family history of suicide, and low concentrations of certain neurotransmitter metabolites (particularly, serotonin metabolite 5-hydroxy-indoleacetic acid (5-HIAA) in cerebrospinal fluid). Anecdotal evidence seems to indicate that among teenagers and young adults, suicide may be influenced by exposure to suicide or suicidal behavior by others. Although this hypothesis has not been formally tested many believe that it warrants recognition and that communities and health officials should have in place a plan to minimize potential contagion before an apparent suicide cluster occurs.

There are a variety of situational risk factors for suicide including stressful life events (e.g., death of a loved one, loss of employment), loss or disruption of normal social support mechanisms (e.g., divorce, moving from one place to another), and absent or inadequate social networks support; these are most dangerous when they interact with other suicide risk factors. Another important situational risk factor is the ready accessibility of firearms. Because a suicide attempt with a firearm is often immediately lethal and very little time is needed to plan for suicide if the firearm is available, suicide with a firearm may be committed impulsively, with little or no time to reconsider the action. Some risk factors for suicide are not "causal" but serve as markers of individuals at high risk: being male, elderly, or having a past history of attempted suicide.

The outcomes of suicide include tremendous economic costs as well as emotional trauma suffered by the family members and friends of the suicide victims. In 1984 suicide of those younger than 65 years of age resulted in a loss of over 645,000 years of potential life. For survivors the emotional trauma is particularly difficult because of the unexpectedness of the event, possible feelings of guilt, the social stigma associated with suicide, and possible withdrawal of the usual social support because of the social stigma.

Interventions for suicide prevention can be divided into five major categories:

1. Improving the identification, referral, and treatment of persons at high risk.
2. Treatment of underlying risk factors, such as clinical depression or alcoholism.
3. Decreasing individual vulnerability to suicide through education of the general population.
4. Making self-referral resources accessible to suicidal persons.

5. Limiting access to lethal means of suicide, such as firearms, prescription drugs, and high places.

A public health priority must be to assess the effectiveness of these interventions so that policy makers can make the best use of limited suicide prevention resources.

STATEMENT OF THE PROBLEM

In 1987 there were 30,796 deaths from suicide in the United States, making suicide the eighth leading cause of death in this country (1). Unlike the rates for many diseases, suicide rates are substantial among both young and old people. As a result, suicide is the fifth leading cause of premature death, as defined by years of potential life lost before age 65 (2). In past decades, the rate of suicide was relatively low among adolescents and young adults but increased steadily with increasing age. However, suicide rates among younger age groups have increased dramatically in the last three to four decades (3). In particular, the suicide rate among persons 15–24 years of age has almost tripled: in 1950 the suicide rate for this age group was 4.5 per 100,000; in 1988, this rate was 12.8 (4,5). Suicide has been the second or third leading cause of death among persons 15–24 years of age in recent years. Although most suicides occur among persons less than forty years of age, the highest rates occur among the elderly (3).

In general, men are three to five times more likely to commit suicide than women. Furthermore, men are at higher risk than women across all age and race groups. White men are at the highest risk of suicide, followed by men of races other than white, white women, and women of races other than white. White men have also experienced the greatest increase in suicide rates among persons 15–24 years of age. In 1987 the rate of suicide in this race-sex-age group was almost twice the overall national suicide rate (6).

For both men and women, firearms are the most frequently used method of suicide; overall, approximately 60 percent of all suicides are committed with firearms. Among men, hanging is the second most common method of suicide, followed by poisoning by gases (chiefly carbon monoxide). Among women, ingestion of an overdose of drugs is the second most common method. The predominance of firearms as a method of suicide is increasing among men, whereas it is new for women. In 1970 for example, more women committed suicide by drug ingestion than by firearms. In recent years, firearm suicides have accounted for an increasingly large proportion of all suicides among persons 15–24 years of age. From 1970 to 1984, the proportion of suicides committed with firearms increased 17 percent and 59 percent for men and women, respectively (7).

Reliable information regarding morbidity from attempted (as opposed to completed) suicide is sparse. In one large, multi-site survey of adults in the

United States, approximately three out of every 1,000 reported having attempted suicide at some point during the preceding year (8). This estimate, which is in line with previous smaller surveys, suggests that approximately 750,000 adults attempt suicide each year in the United States, and that there are approximately 25 suicide attempts for each completed suicide.

DATA SOURCES

Suicide mortality data ultimately derive from death certificate data. The determination of suicide as a cause of death, however, is not always a straightforward process. Suicide has been defined fairly succinctly as death from intentionally self-inflicted injury (9), but it can be very difficult to apply this definition. In particular, determining whether a decedent intended to commit suicide necessarily involves retrospective collection of data regarding the decedent's state of mind prior to the death. The amount and quality of such information varies greatly from case to case. Moreover, until recently there were no published guidelines explicitly describing what type of data ought to be collected in a death investigation in order to make an informed determination of manner of death (9). The great variability across the United States in the qualifications of the coroner or official responsible for medicolegal certification presents additional questions about the validity and reliability of death certificate information (10).

Against the backdrop of these structural problems in suicide certification, there is also the social stigma associated with suicide. For religious, financial, and even political reasons, coroners and medical examiners may sometimes be reluctant to certify suicide as a cause of death. Given these limitations in the way suicide is determined as a cause of death, it is not surprising that many investigators believe official suicide statistics substantially underestimate the true suicide rate. Estimates of the true suicide rate range from a low of 1.01 to 1.8 times the official rate, but it is likely that the true rate of suicide is no more than 1.25 times the offical rate (11).

There is essentially no information at the national level concerning the magnitude of the physical and mental health consequences of attempted suicide. Indeed, the incidence estimates from surveys of adults cited above are quite limited in what they tell us about attempted suicide. Because attempted suicide was self-defined in these surveys, for example, it is unclear what proportion of these "suicide attempts" resulted in injury, in a visit to an emergency health facility, or in subsequent attempted or completed suicide. There are also no national estimates of the incidence of attempted suicide among persons less than 18 years of age, although there are indications that the attempted suicide rate in this group may be even higher than in the adult population. Without such information on a national, longitudinal basis, it is difficult to accurately estimate suicide attempt morbidity and trends, or to assess the efficacy of suicide prevention programs.

CAUSES AND RISK FACTORS

Even though it is common to hear people say that a person committed suicide because he or she was mentally ill or could not cope with stressful events, in reality there are many factors that contribute to the causal mechanism of any given suicide. Certain psychiatric illnesses are, of course, both extremely important and well recognized as risk factors for suicide. In particular, affective disorders have been clearly shown in both retrospective case-control studies and prospective cohort studies to markedly increase the risk of suicide (12). For example, in a population-based cohort study of 3,563 men in Sweden followed for 15 to 25 years, the suicide rate among men with an initial diagnosis of any mental illness was almost 39 times higher than the rate for men with no mental disorder. Men with an initial diagnosis of a depressive disorder had a suicide rate 80 times higher than men with no mental disorder (13).

After clinical depression, alcoholism is the most commonly reported mental illness associated with suicide (14–17). In many studies, however, no control group was used in assessing the contribution of alcohol use to suicide risk (18–20). In addition, the independent effect of alcoholism on the suicide rate is rarely estimated; rather, the diagnosis of alcoholism among the case series is often reported along with the prevalence of affective illness, social isolation, and other factors that might themselves account for any observed increase in the risk of suicide. Most of the studies have been done using special populations, such as psychiatric inpatients (21–23) or hospitalized alcoholics (24–26), and the findings of these studies are not necessarily applicable to alcoholics in general. Finally, very little work has been done to separately assess the effects of acute exposure to alcohol (i.e., alcohol intoxication) and alcohol abuse on the risk of suicide. More research is needed to elucidate the mechanism(s) underlying the observed association between alcoholism and suicide.

Certain personality disorders (in particular, borderline and antisocial personality disorders) have also been shown to be correlated with suicidal behavior (27). The interpretation of this correlation is problematic, however, since suicidal behavior is inherently part of the definition of certain personality disorders, such as borderline personality disorder. The strength and the predictive value of personality disorders as risk factors for suicide, as well as the mechanisms explaining the observed association between certain personality disorders and suicide, must be determined in future research.

There is an increasing body of literature addressing putative genetic and biologic risk factors for suicide. Suicide has long been observed to "run in families," but such a phenomenon might either be caused by common exposure among family members to environmental-sociocultural risk factors for suicide, or by genetic factors shared by family members. Meta-analysis of twin studies, however, strongly suggests a genetically based risk for mental illness and suicide. Moreover, several Danish-American adoption studies suggest that this genetic risk may be inherited independently of major psychiatric illness, perhaps as an inability to control impulsive behavior (28).

Certain neurotransmitter metabolites have been convincingly associated with an increased risk of suicide (29). In particular, a clear relationship has been demonstrated between low concentrations of the serotonin metabolite 5-hydroxyindoleacetic acid (5-HIAA) in cerebrospinal fluid (CSF) and an increased incidence of attempted and completed suicide in psychiatric patients. Most of the evidence for this relationship is based on studies of patients with major affective illness (particularly unipolar depression), but there is some evidence this relationship may hold for other diagnostic categories as well, particularly for personality disorders (30) and possibly for schizophrenia (31). The mechanism that accounts for the relationship between a disturbed or inadequate serotonin system and suicidal behavior is not clear.

Recent suicide clusters among teenagers and young adults have suggested that suicides may sometimes be caused by "contagion," i.e., by exposure to the suicide or suicidal behavior of others (32,33). There is ample anecdotal evidence to suggest that, in any given suicide cluster, suicides occurring later in the cluster often appear to have been influenced by suicides occurring earlier in the cluster (34,35). This contagion hypothesis has never been formally tested at the individual level, and the strength and public health importance of contagion as a risk factor for suicide remain to be determined. In general, contagion in the context of suicide clusters has been conceptualized as being mediated through an amalgam of imitation, identification, grief, and the highly charged emotional atmosphere common in many communities that have experienced suicide clusters. Despite uncertainty about contagion as a risk factor for suicide, many believe it is prudent to recognize the possibility of a contagious effect of suicide and to institute measures to minimize potential contagion in the context of an apparent suicide cluster (36).

Suicide contagion may not be limited to geographically localized clusters of suicides. A number of ecologic studies have been done to assess whether the incidence of suicide in the general population is increased by exposure to television news stories and movies about suicide. Some investigators have reported an increase in suicide following such exposure (37,38), but this finding has not been found in all studies (39,40) and has been challenged in others (41,42). Both the nature of the exposure to suicide and the hypothesized induction period from exposure to outcome in these studies are quite different than is hypothesized for geographically localized suicide clusters. In the former, the exposure is to stories, fictional or otherwise, of suicides by persons unknown to the study subjects; the induction period implied in the study designs is one to two weeks. In the case of geographically localized suicide clusters, however, the suicides to which victims of the suicide cluster were exposed were frequently those of close or intimate friends; reported suicide clusters have typically occurred over the course of one to four months (43), but have ranged from several weeks to over one year (44).

There are a variety of situational risk factors for suicide. Stressful life events, such as the death of a loved one or recent loss of employment, often appear to be clear precipitants of suicide (45). In general, stressful life events may elevate the background risk of suicide by a factor of five to 10, although the duration of time after exposure to these stressful events during which suicide risk remains elevated has not been well characterized (46). A loss or disruption of normal social support mechanisms also increases the risk of suicide. Divorce, unemployment, and migration from one community to another are but three examples of factors that may lead to some disruption of social support networks; all three have been shown to be related to increased suicide rates (12,47). Absent or inadequate social support networks presumably increase the risk of suicide through interaction with other suicide risk factors, such as clinical depression and recent stressful life events.

Another situational risk factor of potentially great importance is the ready accessibility of firearms. Unlike drug ingestions, carbon monoxide poisoning, and many other suicide methods, a suicide attempt with a firearm is often immediately lethal, leaving little or no opportunity for post-attempt rescue. Moreover, if a firearm is readily accessible, very little planning and time are required between the moment a person decides to commit suicide and the execution of the attempt. The accessibility of a firearm may both limit the preattempt opportunity for intervention by others and facilitate impulsive suicidal acts (48,49). Theoretically, at least some proportion of impulsive decisions to commit suicide might never be acted on if substantial efforts were necessary to arrange for a suicide method. However, the factors that determine choice of suicide method are complex, and careful research is needed to determine whether accessibility to firearms increases the risk of suicide.

Finally, there are several risk factors for suicide that are useful for delineating high risk groups, although these factors do not appear to be "causal" in the traditional sense. Being male, for example, or being elderly, identifies one as belonging to a high risk group. Having a past history of attempted suicide has also been clearly shown to increase the risk of future completed suicide (12). These markers for increased suicide risk presumably correlate with other, causal risk factors for suicide. A past history of attempted suicide, for example, may correlate with impulsivity or with a vulnerability to affective illness.

OUTCOMES

In human and economic terms, the cost of suicide in the United States is enormous. In 1984 alone, suicide among those younger than 65 years of age resulted in the loss of over 645,000 years of potential life (50). Weinstein and Saturno (51) estimate that in 1980, suicide among persons 15–24 years of age alone resulted in the loss of 276,000 years of potential life and economic costs of $2.26 billion. Adding in attempted suicide among persons in this age group brought the estimated economic costs to $3.19 billion.

The emotional trauma experienced by the "survivors" of suicide—family members and friends of suicide victims—is enormous (52). The process of grief and bereavement over the death of a loved one is always painful and difficult, but when the decedent committed suicide, this process is even more difficult and traumatic. Death from suicide is usually sudden and unexpected. Suicide may engender feelings of guilt or rejection in the survivors. Because of the social stigma associated with suicide, traditional mourning rituals may be avoided, and the usual social supports for the decedent's family and friends may be withdrawn or attenuated. All of these factors increase the risk of disturbed or unresolved grief reactions among the survivors (53).

INTERVENTIONS

Although a wide variety of suicide prevention programs have been devised, the strategies underlying these programs may be considered under five broad conceptual categories. The first such strategy is to improve the identification, referral, and treatment of persons at high risk of suicide by various caretakers and "gatekeepers" in the community. Increased training of primary care physicians in the recognition and treatment or referral of patients with clinical depression is one example of this approach; school-based screening programs designed to identify suicidal youth in the context of an evolving suicide cluster is another. A second suicide prevention strategy focuses on the treatment of underlying risk factors for suicide. Clinical depression, for example, is addressed through psychotherapeutic and pharmacologic treatment of patients with this illness. Alcohol rehabilitation programs, though not traditionally thought of in terms of suicide prevention, may contribute to the prevention of suicide by addressing one of the most important risk factors for suicide—alcoholism.

A third general suicide prevention strategy is to decrease individual vulnerability to suicide through education of the general population. Affective education programs, for example, seek to help individuals understand and cope with the types of problems that can lead to suicide (54). Other programs are designed to increase public awareness of helping resources in the community to facilitate help-seeking behavior by suicidal persons. A fourth, related suicide prevention strategy is to provide or expand the accessibility of self-referral resources for suicidal persons. Hot lines and walk-in crisis centers are the best-known examples of this strategy.

A final strategy for suicide prevention seeks to limit access to lethal means of suicide, such as high places, prescription drugs, or firearms (55). This strategy derives from the hypothesis that if substantial efforts are required by an individual to arrange for a lethal suicide method, of if a less lethal method is substituted in its stead, the likelihood of a completed suicide will be diminished.

The above strategies have differing strengths and weaknesses, and each may be important in the prevention of suicide. Unfortunately, the effectiveness of many of these strategies has yet to be established. Eddy and colleagues (54) surveyed 15 suicide experts as to their judgments of the effectiveness of a variety of existing and proposed youth suicide prevention strategies. On the average, these experts estimated that approximately 10 percent of potential youth suicides were being averted by existing prevention programs, and that each of the proposed strategies to improve prevention might reduce the incidence of youth suicide by 6–16 percent, depending on the strategy. Even if all of the proposed strategies were simultaneously implemented, the expected reduction in youth suicide was estimated to range from 15 percent to no more than 50 percent. The uncertainty regarding program effectiveness, and the relatively modest nature of the reduction in mortality that may be expected from our present array of interventions, is not limited to youth suicide prevention programs but extends to suicide prevention in general. There is clearly an urgent need to develop a better empirical base of information regarding the effectiveness of various prevention strategies so that policy makers can make the best use of limited suicide prevention resources.

Approaching Suicide as a Public Health Problem

As we move from continuing research on risk factors and evaluating strategies to actually developing programs and interventions, it is important to consider the role of public health in suicide prevention and how the multisectorial collaboration necessary for successful suicide prevention program can be achieved. It is important to emphasize that suicide be addressed as a public health problem and not solely a mental health problem.

Suicide is not Solely Determined by Mental Illness

Mental illness is not the only relevant risk factor in the causal mechanism leading to suicide. Research has consistently pointed to the importance of many other factors unrelated to mental illness as important determinants of suicide such as accessibility to firearms, geographic mobility, parental loss, family disruption, being a friend or family member of a suicide victim, alcohol and drug use, and social isolation. If suicide prevention efforts focus solely on mental illness and ignore the contribution of other factors that contribute to suicide, many lives may be lost that could otherwise have been saved.

For Those Suicides for which Mental Illness is the Key Risk Factor, It is Inappropriate to Confine Prevention Efforts to the Mental Health Sector

Mental health practitioners can only accomplish the important clinical work they do when patients come to see them. There are many factors, however, that determine whether suicidal patients seek help from mental health professionals. The most striking example of progress in this area is the training of "gatekeepers" across a variety of disciplines (e.g., education, general medicine). These gatekeepers often play a critical role in facilitating proper care by mental health professionals—but training these gatekeepers is a task that is in large part beyond the scope of mental health systems.

An Effective Approach to Suicide Prevention Requires
the Collaboration of Individuals in Public Health,
Mental Health, Medicine, Education, and Social Services
in Both the Public and Private Sector
One of the most important developments in the field of suicidology in the last 30 years has been the recognition that suicide prevention cannot be accomplished solely through the efforts of one societal sector. This realization was clearly recognized by the Secretary's Task Force on Youth Suicide and highlighted among the major recommendations of this body. The characterization of suicide itself as directly a mental health problem (as opposed to depression, for example, which is an important risk factor for suicide) undermine efforts to engender multidisciplinary and intersectorial efforts to prevent suicide.

Although Mental Illness is an Important Risk Factor
for Suicide Across All Age Groups, Mental Illness Plays
its Least Important Role in the Etiology of the Suicide among
Youth Ages 15-24, the Group in which Suicide Rates
have been Increasing Most Rapidly.
Research conducted by David Shaffer and his colleagues has shown that mental illness, particularly depression, a common antecedent to suicide in adults, may be less frequently associated with suicide among young people (personal communication). In fact, Shaffer has concluded that uncomplicated depression, without any associated behavior problems, is uncommon among youths who commit suicide and that only a small proportion of teen suicides occur among teenagers with manic depressive or schizophrenic psychosis because these conditions are relatively rare. Consequently, prevention strategies that focus on mental illness would appear to be insufficient for the prevention of youth suicide.

For These Reasons, State and Local Public Health Agencies
and other Interested Groups Should Play Key Roles
in Suicide Prevention Efforts
Mental health professionals and mental health agencies have a large and very important role to play in suicide prevention; however, their efforts will be enhanced by a broader view of the nature of suicide and how we may best prevent it.

REFERENCES

1. National Center for Health Statistics. Advance report of final mortality statistics, 1987. Hyattsville, Maryland: Public Health Service, 1989; DHHS publication no. (PHS)89-1120. (Monthly Vital Statistics Report; vol 38, no 5 supp).
2. Centers for Disease Control. Premature mortality due to suicide and homicide—United States, 1983. MMWR 1986; 35:357–365.
3. Rosenberg ML, Smith JC, Davidson LE, Conn JM. The emergence of youth suicide: An epidemiologic analysis and public health perspective. Annu Rev Public Health 1987; 8:417–440.
4. Centers for Disease Control. Youth suicide in the United States, 1970–1980. Atlanta: Centers for Disease Control, 1986.
5. National Center for Health Statistics. Annual summary of births, marriages, divorces, and deaths: United States, 1988. Monthly Vital Statistics Report 1989; 37(13):21.
6. National Center for Health Statistics, unpublished final data. Table 290: Death rates for 72 selected causes, by 10-year age groups, color, and sex: United States, 1979–87, pp. 486, 488.
7. Saltzman LE, Levenson A, Smith JA. Suicides among persons 15–24 years of age, 1970–1984. In: Centers for Disease Control. CDC Surveillance Summaries, February 1988. MMWR 1988;37 (No. SS-1): 61–68.
8. Moscicki EK, O'Carroll PW, Rae DS, Roy AG, Locke BZ, Regier DA. Suicidal ideation and attempts: The Epidemiologic Catchment Area study. In: Alcohol, Drug Abuse and Mental Health Administration. Report of the Secretary's Task Force on Youth Suicide. Volume 4: Strategies for the prevention of youth suicide. DHHS Pub. No. (ADM)89-1624. Washington, DC: US Govt. Printing Office, 1989: 115–128.
9. Rosenberg ML, Davidson LE, Smith JC, Berman AL, Buzbee H, Gantner G, Gay GA, Moore-Lewis B, Mills DH, Murray D, O'Carroll PW, Jobes D. Operational criteria for the determination of suicide. J Forensic Sci 1988; 33:1445–1456.
10. Nelson FL, Farberow NL, MacKinnon DR. The certification of suicide in eleven Western states: An inquiry into the validity of reported suicide rates. Suicide Life-Threat Behav 1978; 8:75–88.
11. O'Carroll PW. A consideration of the validity and reliability of suicide mortality data. Suicide Life-Threat Behav 1989; 19:1–16.
12. Monk M. Epidemiology of suicide. Epidemiol Rev 1987; 9:51–69.
13. Hagnell O, Lanke J, Rorsman B. Suicide rates in the Lundby study: Mental illness as a risk factor for suicide. Neuropsychobiology 1981; 7:248–253.
14. Murphy GE. Problems in studying suicide. Psychiatr Dev 1983; 1(4):339–350.
15. Miles CP. Conditions predisposing to suicide: A review. J Nerv Ment Dis 1977; 164(4):231–246.
16. Roy A, Linnoila M. Alcoholism and suicide. Suicide Life-Threat Behav 1986; 16(2):244–273.
17. Kendall RE. Alcohol and suicide. Subst Alcohol Actions Misuse 1983; 4(2–3):121–127.
18. Fernandez-Pol B. Characteristics of 77 Puerto Ricans who attempted suicide. Am J Psychiatry 1986; 143(11):1460–1463.
19. Kost-Grant BL. Self-inflicted gunshot wounds among Alaska Natives. Public Health Rep 1983 Jan–Feb; 98(1):72–78.

20. Chynoweth R, Tonge JI, Armstrong J. Suicide in Brisbane—a retrospective psychosocial study. Aust NZ J Psychiatry 1980; 14(1):37–45.
21. Morrison JR. Suicide in a psychiatric practice population. J Clin Psychiatry 1982; 43(9):348–352.
22. Robbins DR, Alessi NE. Depressive symptoms and suicidal behavior in adolescents. Am J Psychiatry 1985; 142(5):588–592.
23. Black DW, Warrack G, Winokur G. The Iowa record-linkage study. I. Suicides and accidental deaths among psychiatric patients. Arch Gen Psychiatry 1985; 42(1):71–75.
24. Shuckitt MA. Primary men alcoholics with histories of suicide attempts. J Stud Alcohol 1986; 47(1):78–81.
25. Bacue LO, Epstein L. Suicide attitudes and experiences of hospitalized alcoholics. Psychol Rep 1980; 47(3 Pt 2):1233–1234.
26. Berglund M. Suicide in alcoholism. A prospective study of 88 suicides: I. The multidimensional diagnosis at first admission. Arch Gen Psychiatry 1984; 41(9):888–891.
27. Frances A, Blumenthal S. Personality as a predictor of youthful suicide. In: Alcohol, Drug Abuse and Mental Health Administration. Report of the Secretary's Task Force on Youth Suicide. Vol. 2: Risk factors for youth suicide. DHHS Pub. No. (ADM)89-1624. Washington, DC: US Govt. Printing Office, 1989: 160–171.
28. Roy A. Genetics and suicidal behavior. In: Alcohol, Drug Abuse and Mental Health Administration. Report of the Secretary's Task Force on Youth Suicide. Vol. 2: Risk factors for youth suicide. DHHS Pub. No. (ADM)89-1624. Washington, DC: US Govt. Printing Office, 1989: 247–262.
29. Asberg M. Neurotransmitter monoamine metabolites in the cerebrospinal fluid as risk factors for suicidal behavior. In: Alcohol, Drug Abuse and Mental Health Administration. Report of the Secretary's Task Force on Youth Suicide. Vol. 2: Risk factors for youth suicide. DHHS Pub. No. (ADM)89-1624. Washington, DC: US Govt. Printing Office, 1989: 193–212.
30. Traskman L, Asberg M, Bertillson L, Sjostrand L. Monoamine metabolites in CSF and suicidal behavior. Arch Gen Psychiatry 1981; 38:631–636.
31. van Praag HM. CSF 5-HIAA and suicide in non-depressed schizophrenics. Lancet 1983; 2:977–978.
32. Robbins D, Conroy C. A cluster of adolescent suicide attempts: Is suicide contagious? J Adolesc Health Care 1983; 3:253–255.
33. Davidson L, Gould MS. Contagion as a risk factor for youth suicide. In: Alcohol, Drug Abuse, and Mental Health Administration. Report of the Secretary's Task Force on Youth Suicide. Vol. 2: Risk factors for youth suicide. DHHS Pub. No. (ADM)89-1622. Washington, DC: US Govt. Printing Office, 1989: 88–109.
34. Centers for Disease Control. Cluster of suicides and suicide attempts—New Jersey. MMWR 1988; 37:213–216.
35. O'Carroll PW. An investigation of a cluster of suicide attempts. In: Yufit RI, ed. Combined proceedings of the twentieth annual meeting of the American Association of Suicidology and the nineteenth annual congress of the International Association of Suicide Prevention. San Francisco: American Association of Suicidology, 1987: 262–264.
36. O'Carroll PW, Mercy JA, Steward JA. CDC Recommendations for a community plan for the prevention and containment of suicide clusters. MMWR 1988; 37 (suppl. no. S-6):1–12.

37. Phillips DP, Carstensen LL. Clustering of teenage suicides after television news stories about suicide. N Engl J Med 1986; 315:685–689.
38. Gould MS, Shaffer D. The impact of suicide in television movies: Evidence of imitation. N Engl J Med 1986; 315:690–694.
39. Phillips DP, Paight DJ. The impact of televised movies about suicide: A replicative study. N Engl J Med 1987; 317:809–811.
40. Berman AL. Fictional depiction of suicide in television films and imitation effects. Am J Psychiatry 1988; 145:982–986.
41. Kessler RC, Stipp H. The impact of fictional television suicide stories on U.S. fatalities: A replication. Am J Sociology 1984; 90:151–167.
42. Baron JN, Reiss PC. Same time, next year: Aggregate analyses of the mass media and violent behavior. Am Sociol Rev 1985; 50:347–363.
43. Gould MS. A study of time-space clustering. Phase I Report. Atlanta: Centers for Disease Control, 1985 (Contract No. RFP 200-85-0834).
44. Davidson LE, Rosenberg ML, Mercy JA, et al. An epidemiologic study of risk factors in two teenage suicide clusters. JAMA 1989; 262:2687–2692.
45. See, for example, Paykel ES, Prusoff BA, Myers JK. Suicide attempts and recent life events: A controlled comparison. Arch Gen Psychiatry 1975; 32:327–337.
46. Paykel ES. Stress and life events. In: Alcohol, Drug Abuse and Mental Health Administration. Report of the Secretary's Task Force on Youth Suicide. Vol. 2: Risk factors for youth suicide. DHHS Pub. No. (ADM)89-1624. Washington, DC: US Govt. Printing Office, 1989: 110–130.
47. Platt S. Unemployment and suicidal behavior: A review of the literature. Soc Sci Med 1984; 19:93–115.
48. Boyd JH. The increasing rate of suicide by firearms. N Engl J Med 1983; 308:872–874.
49. Sloan JH, Rivara FP, Reay DT, Ferris JAJ, Kellerman AL. Firearm regulations and rates of suicide: A comparison of two metropolitan areas. N Engl J Med 1990; 322:369–373.
50. Centers for Disease Control. Premature mortality due to suicide and homicide—United States, 1984. MMWR 1987; 36:531–534.
51. Weinstein MC, Saturno PJ. Economic impact of youth suicides and suicide attempts. In: Alcohol, Drug Abuse and Mental Health Administration. Report of the Secretary's Task Force on Youth Suicide. Vol. 4: Strategies for the prevention of youth suicide. DHHS Pub. No. (ADM)89-1624. Washington, DC: US Govt. Printing Office, 1989: 82–93.
52. Dunne EJ, Dunne-Maxim K. Suicide and its aftermath: Understanding and counseling the survivors. New York: W.W. Norton, 1987.
53. Hauser MJ. Special aspects of grief after a suicide. In: Dunne EJ, Dunne-Maxim K, eds. Suicide and its aftermath: Understanding and counseling the survivors. New York: W.W. Norton, 1987: 57–70.
54. Eddy DM, Wolpert RL, Rosenberg ML. Estimating the effectiveness of interventions to prevent youth suicides. In: Alcohol, Drug Abuse and Mental Health Administration. Report of the Secretary's Task Force on Youth Suicide. Vol. 4: Strategies for the prevention of youth suicide. DHHS Pub. No. (ADM)89-1624. Washington, DC: US Govt. Printing Office, 1989: 37–81.
55. The National Committee for Injury Prevention and Control. Injury prevention: Meeting the challenge. New York: Oxford University Press, 1989: 252–260.

Index